THE
VITAMIN
BIBLE

THE VITAMIN BIBLE

*How the right vitamins
and nutrient supplements
can revolutionise your life*

Earl Mindell

*Arlington Books
King Street, St. James's
London S.W.1*

THE VITAMIN BIBLE
First published 1979 in the United States of America
This edition first published September 1982 in England by
Arlington Books (Publishers) Ltd, London

Distributed by Biblios Ltd, Horsham

Reprinted 1982
Reprinted four times 1983
Reprinted 1984
Second Edition (revised and expanded)
First published June 1985
Reprinted 1985, 1986, 1987 (twice),
1988 (twice), 1989 (twice),
1990, 1991, 1992, 1993

Typeset by Inforum Ltd, Portsmouth
Printed and bound in Great Britain by
Biddles Ltd, Guildford and King's Lynn

British Library Cataloguing in Publication Data
Mindell, Earl
The vitamin bible: how the right vitamins and
nutrient supplements can revolutionise your
life.—New ed.
1. Vitamins   2. Vitamins in human nutrition
I. Title   II. Mindell, Earl, Earl Mindell's
vitamin bible
613.2'8   QP771

ISBN 0–85140–672–6

This book is dedicated to
Gail, Alanna, Evan,
our parents and families
and to the future

"The first wealth is health."
Ralph Waldo Emerson
The Conduct of Life

Acknowledgments

I wish to express my deep and lasting appreciation to my friends and associates who have assisted me in the preparation of this book, especially J. Kenney, Ph.D.; Linus Pauling, Ph.D.; Hester Mundis; Bernard Bubman, R.Ph.; and Mel Rich, R.Ph.

I would also like to thank the Nutrition Foundation; the International College of Applied Nutrition; the American Medical Association; the New York Blood Centre; the American Academy of Paediatrics; the American Dietetic Association; the National Academy of Sciences; the National Dairy Council; the Society for Nutrition Association; the United Fresh Fruit and Vegetable Association; the Albany College of Pharmacy; Peter Mallory; Edward Leavitt, D.V.M.; Debbi Quick; Ronald Borenstein; Laura Borenstein; Martha Millard and Richard Curtis, without whom a project of this scope could never have been completed.

A note to the reader about this newly revised 2nd edition

Since the first publication of *The Vitamin Bible* in 1979, the field of vitamins and nutrition has exploded. More people than ever before in history are taking supplements, and startling new discoveries about the interrelation between vitamins, drugs, natural foods, and health are being made daily. Preventive medicine is no longer a fad, but a fact — as attested to by the conservative National Academy of Sciences' recent report that 80–85% of all human internal cancers could be prevented through improved nutrition.

Other new discoveries, such as how the right foods and supplements can effectively substitute for drugs, alleviate the discomforts of premenstrual syndrome (PMS), rejuvenate the metabolism, improve the immune system, reduce the risk of heart disease, act as natural pain-killers, fatigue reducers, and much more, are included in this new expanded edition, along with complete new sections on amino acids, herbs, and the latest cautions about them all.

Preface

This book is written for *you* — the untold legions of men and women who are forever trying to fit yourselves into statistical norms only to find that the charts are designed for some mythical average person who is taller, shorter, fatter, skinnier, less or more active than you'll ever be. It is a guide to healthy living for individuals, not statistics. Wherever feasible, I have given personal advice, for this, I believe, is the only way to lead anyone to optimum health, which is the purpose of this book.

In these pages I have combined my knowledge of pharmacy with that of nutrition to best explain the confusing, often dangerous, interrelation of drugs and vitamins. I've attempted to be specific so as to eliminate much of the confusion about vitamins that has arisen with generalisations.

In using the book you will occasionally find that your vitamin needs fall into several different categories. In this case, let common sense dictate the necessary adjustment. [If you are already taking B_2, for example, there's no need to double up on it unless a higher dosage is called for.]

The recommendations I've made are not meant to be prescriptive, but can easily be used as flexible programmes *when working with your doctor. No book can substitute for professional care.*

My professional education was strictly establishment when it came to vitamins. My courses in pharmacology, biochemistry, organic and inorganic chemistry, and public health hardly dealt with vitamins at all — except in relation to deficiency diseases.

There were no references to vitamins being used for disease prevention or as ways to optimum health.

In 1965 I opened my first pharmacy. Until then I never realised how many drugs people were taking, not for illness but simply to get through the day. My partner at the time was very vitamin-oriented. Both of us were working fifteen hours a day, but only *I* looked and felt it. When I asked him what his secret was, he said it was no secret at all. It was vitamins. After embarking on the most elementary vitamin regimens I was not only convinced. I was converted.

Suddenly nutrition became the most important thing in my life. I read every book I could find on the subject, clipped articles and tracked down their sources, dug out my pharmacy school texts and discovered the amazingly close relationship that did exist between biochemistry and nutrition. I attended any health lecture I could. [It was at once such lecture that I learned of the RNA–DNA nucleic complex and its age-reversing properties. I have been taking RNA–DNA supplements since then, and today most people guess me to be five to ten years younger than I am.] I was excited about each new discovery in the field, and it showed.

By 1970 I was totally committed to nutrition and preventive medicine. Seeing the paucity of knowledge in the area, I went into partnership with another pharmacist for the prime purpose of making natural vitamins and accurate nutrition information available to the public.

Today, as a nutritionist, lecturer, and author, I'm still excited about that world that opened up to me over fifteen years ago — a world that continues to grow with new discoveries daily — and I'm eager to share it.

It is my sincerest hope that I have provided you with information that will help you attain the longest, happiest, and healthiest of lives.

EARL MINDELL, *Pharm.B., R.Ph.*

One important reminder

The regimens throughout this book are recommendations, not prescriptions, and are not intended as medical advice. Before starting any new programme check with your physician or a nutritionally oriented doctor, especially if you have a specific physical problem, or are taking any medication.

Contents

PART ONE

THE WHOLE TRUTH

What vitamins are — What vitamins are not — How they work — Should you take supplements — *What are nutrients?* — The difference between micronutrients and macronutrients — How nutrients get to work — Understanding your digestive system — Name that vitamin — Name that mineral — Your body needs Vitamins and Minerals

Where vitamins come from — Why vitamins come in different forms — Oil vs. dry or water soluble — Synthetic vs. natural and inorganic vs. organic — Chelation, and what it means – Time release — Fillers, binders, or what else are you getting? — Storage and staying power — When and how to take supplements — What's right for you

Vitamin A — Vitamin B_1 [Thiamine] — Vitamin B_2 [Riboflavin]

— Vitamin B_6 [Pyridoxine] — Vitamin B_{12} [Cobalamin] — Vitamin B_{13} [Orotic Acid]— Vitamin B_{15} [Pangamic Acid] — Vitamin B_{17} [Laetrile] — Biotin [Coenzyme R or Vitamin H] — Vitamin C [Ascorbic Acid, Cevitamin Acid] — Calcium Pantothenate [Pantothenic Acid, Panthenol, Vitamin B_5] — Choline — Vitamin D [Calciferol, Viosterol, Ergosterol, "Sunshine Vitamin"] — Vitamin E [Tocopherol] — Vitamin F [Unsaturated Fatty Acids — Linoleic, Arachidonic]— Folic Acid [Folacin] — Inositol — Vitamin K [Menadione] — Niacin [Nicotinic Acid, Niacinamide, Nicotinamide] — Vitamin P [C Complex, Citrus Bioflavonoids, Rutin, Hesperidin] — PABA [Para-aminobenzoic Acid] — Vitamin T — Vitamin U that measure up? — What's what in weights and measures — Breaking the RDA code — What to look for

PART TWO

GETTING YOURS

Arthritis — Blood pressure — hight and low — Bronchitis — Chicken pox — Colds — Colitis — Diabetes — Eye problems — Heart conditions — Hypoglycaemia — Impetigo — Measles — Mononucleosis — Mumps — Shingles — Tonsilitis — Ulcers — Venereal disease

11

PART ONE

THE
WHOLE TRUTH

I

Getting into Vitamins

What Vitamins Are

We must obtain vitamins from organic foods, or dietary supplements in order to sustain life. When I mention the word "vitamin", most people think "pill". Thinking "pill" brings to mind confusing images of medicine and drugs. Though vitamins can and certainly often do the work of both medicine and drugs, they are neither.

Quite simply, vitamins are organic substances necessary for life. Vitamins are essential to the normal functioning of our bodies and, save for a few exceptions, cannot be manufactured or synthesised by our bodies. They are necessary for our growth, vitality, and general well-being. In their natural state they are found in minute quantities in all organic food. We must obtain them from these foods or in dietary supplements.

Supplements, which usually come in pill form and around which so much controversy has arisen, are still just food substances, and, unless synthetic, are also derived from living plants and animals.

It is impossible to sustain life without *all* the essential vitamins.

What Vitamins are Not

Vitamins are neither pep pills nor substitutes for food. A lot of people think vitamins can replace food. They cannot. In fact, vitamins cannot be assimilated without ingesting food. There are a lot of erroneous beliefs about vitamins, and I hope this book can clear up most of them.

Vitamins are not pep pills and have no caloric or energy value of their own.

15

Vitamins are not substitutes for protein or for any other nutrients, such as minerals, fats, carbohydrates, water — or even for each other!

Vitamins themselves are not the components of our body structures.

You cannot take vitamins, stop eating, and expect to be healthy.

How they Work

If you think of the body as a car's combustion engine and vitamins as spark plugs, you have a fairly good idea of how these amazing minute food substances work for us. Vitamins regulate our metabolism through enzyme systems. A single deficiency can endanger the whole body. Vitamins are components of our enzyme systems which, acting like spark plugs, energise and regulate our metabolism, keeping us tuned up and functioning at high performance.

Compared with our intake of other nutrients like proteins, fats, and carbohydrates, our vitamin intake [even on some megadose regimens] is minuscule. But a deficiency in even one vitamin can endanger the whole human body.

Should You Take Supplements?

Since vitamins occur in all organic material, some containing more of one vitamin than another and in greater or lesser amounts, you could say that if you ate the "right" foods in a well-balanced diet, you would get all the vitamins you need. And you would probably be right. The problem is, very few of us are able to arrange this mythical diet. According to Dr. Daniel T. Quigley, author of *The National Malnutrition*, "Everyone who has in the past eaten sugar, white flour, or canned food has some deficiency disease, the extent of the disease depending on the percentage of such deficient food in the diet."

Most of the foods we eat have been processed and depleted in nutrients. Take breads and cereals, for example, Practically all of them you find in today's supermarkets are high in nothing but carbohydrates. "But they are enriched!" you say. It says so right on the label. *Enriched.*

Enriched? The standard of enrichment for white flour is to replace the twenty-two natural nutrients that are removed with three B vitamins, vitamin D, calcium, and iron salts. For the staff of life, that seems a pretty flimsy stick. I think the answer on supplements is clear.

What Are Nutrients?

They're more than vitamins, though people often think they are the same thing.

The six important nutrients are carbohydrates, proteins, fats, minerals, vitamins, and water —absorbable components of foods — and necessary for good health. Nutrients are necessary for energy, organ function, food utilisation, and cell growth.

The Difference Between Micronutrients and Macronutrients

Micronutrients, like vitamins and minerals, do not themselves provide energy. The macronutrients — carbohydrates, fat and protein — do that, but only when there are sufficient micronutrients to release them. With nutrients, *less* is often the same as *more.* The amount of micronutrients and macronutrients you need for proper health is vastly different — but each is important.

How Nutrients Get to Work

The body simplifies nutrients in order to utilise them. Nutrients basically work through digestion. Digestion is a process of continuous chemical simplication of materials that enter the body through the mouth. Materials are split by enzymatic action into smaller and simpler chemical fragments, which can then be absorbed through walls of the digestive tract — an open-ended muscular tube, more than thirty feet long, which passes through the body — and finally enter the bloodstream.

Understanding Your Digestive System

Knowing how your digestive system works will clear up, right at the start, some of the more common confusions about how, when, and where nutrients operate.

Mouth and Oesophagus   Digestion begins in the mouth with the grinding of food and admixture of saliva. An enzyme called ptyalin in the saliva already begins to split starches into simple sugars. The food is then forced to the back of the mouth and into the oesophagus, or gullet. Here is where peristalsis begins. This is a kneading "milking" constriction and relaxation of muscles that propels material through the digestive system. To prevent back-flow of materials, and to time the release of proper enzymes — since one enzyme cannot do another enzyme's work — the digestive tract is equipped with valves at important junctions.

Stomach   This is the biggest bulge in the digestive tract, as most of us are well aware. But it is located higher than you might think, lying mainly behind the lower ribs, not under the navel, and it does not occupy the belly. It is a flexible bag enclosed by restless muscles, constantly changing form. Virtually nothing is absorbed through the stomach walls except alcohol.

An ordinary meal leaves the stomach in three to five hours. Watery substances, such as soup, leave the stomach quite rapidly. Fats remain considerably longer. An ordinary meal of carbohydrates, proteins, and fats is emptied from the average stomach in *three* to *five* hours. Stomach glands and specialised cells produce mucous enzymes, hydrochloric acid, and a factor that enables vitamin B_{12} to be dissolved through intestinal walls into the circulation. A normal stomach is definitely on the acid side, and gastric juice, the stomach's special blend, consists of many substances:

Pepsin   The predominant stomach enzyme, a potent digester of meats and other proteins, it is active only in an acid medium.
Renin   Curdles milk.
HCl [*Hydrochloric acid*]   Produced by stomach cells and creates an acidic state.

The stomach is not absolutely indispensable to digestion. Most of the process of digestion occurs beyond it.

18

Small Intestine Virtually all absorption of nutrients occurs in the small intestine. Twenty-two feet long, here is where digestion is completed and virtually all absorption of nutrients occurs. It has an alkaline environment, brought about by highly alkaline bile, pancreatic juice, and secretions of the intestinal walls. The alkaline environment is necessary for the most important work of digestion and absorption. The *duodenum*, which begins at the stomach outlet, is the first part of the small intestine. This joins with the *jejunum* [about ten feet long], which joins with the *ileum* [ten to twelve feet long]. When semi-liquid contents of the small intestine are moved along by peristaltic action, we often say we hear our stomach "talking". Actually our stomach lies above these rumblings [called borborygmi], but even with the truth known it's doubtful the phrase will change.

Large intestine or Colon It takes twelve to fourteen hours for contents to make the circuit of the large intestine. Any material leaving the ileum and entering the caecum [where the small and large intestines join] is quite watery. Backflow is prevented at this junction by a muscular valve.

Very little is absorbed from the large intestine except water.

The colon is primarily a storage and dehydrating organ. Substances entering in a liquid state become semi-solid as water is absorbed.

The colon, in contrast to the germ-free stomach, is lavishly populated with bacteria, normal intestinal flora. A large part of the faeces is composed of bacteria, along with indigestible material, chiefly cellulose, and substances eliminated from the blood and shed from the intestinal walls.

Liver The main storage organ for fat-soluble vitamins. The liver is the largest solid organ of the body and weighs about four pounds. It is an incomparable chemical plant. It can modify almost any chemical structure. It is a powerful detoxifying organ, breaking down a variety of toxic molecules and rendering them harmless. It is also a blood reservoir and a storage organ for vitamins such as A and D and for digested carbohydrate [glycogen], which is released to sustain blood sugar levels. It manufactures enzymes, cholesterol, proteins, vitamin A [from

19

carotene], and blood coagulation factors.

One of the prime functions of the liver is to produce bile. Bile contains salts that promote efficient digestion of fats by detergent action, emulsifying fatty materials.

Gallbladder   Even the sight of food may empty the gallbladder. This is a sack-like storage organ about three inches long. It holds bile, modifies it chemically, and concentrates it tenfold. The taste or sometimes even the sight of food may be sufficient to empty it out. Constituents of gallbladder fluids sometimes crystallise and form gallstones.

Pancreas   The pancreas provides the body's most important enzymes. This gland is about six inches long, and is nestled into the curve of the duodenum. Its cell clusters secrete insulin, which accelerates the burning of sugar in the body. Insulin is secreted into the blood, not the digestive tract. The larger part of the pancreas manufactures and secretes pancreatic juice, which contains some of the body's most important digestive enzymes — *lipases*, which split fats; *proteases*, which split protein; and *amylases*, which split starches.

Name That Vitamin

Because at one time no one knew the chemical structure of vitamins and therefore could not give them a proper scientific name, most are designated by a letter of the alphabet. The following vitamins are known today; many more have yet to be discovered. A [retinol, carotene]; B-complex group: B_1 [thiamine], B_2[riboflavin], B_3 [niacin, niacinamide], B_5 [pantothenic acid], B_6 [pyridoxine], B_{10}, B_{11}, [growth factors], B_{12} [cobalamine, cyano-cobalamine], B_{13} [orotic acid], B_{15} [pangamic acid], B_{17} [amygdalin]; PABA [para-aminobenzoic acid]; choline; inositol; C [ascorbic acid]; D [calciferol, viosterol, ergosterol]; E [tocopherol]; F [fatty acids]; G [riboflavin]; H [biotin]; K [menadione]; L [necessary for lactation]; M [folic acid]; P [bioflavonoids]; T [growth-promoting substances]; U [extracted from cabbage juice].

Name That Mineral

The top six minerals are: calcium, iodine, iron, magnesium, phosphorus, and zinc. Although about eighteen known minerals are required for body maintenance and regulatory functions, Recommended Daily Dietary Allowances (RDA) have only been established for six — calcium, iodine, iron, magnesium, phosphorus, and zinc.

The active minerals in your body are: calcium, chlorine, chromium, cobalt, copper, fluorine, iodine, iron, magnesium, manganese, molybdenum, phosphorus, potassium, selenium, sodium, sulphur, vanadium, and zinc.

Your Body Needs Vitamins *and* Minerals

Vitamins alone are not enough. As important as vitamins are, they can do nothing for you without minerals. I like to call minerals the Cinderellas of the nutrition world, because though very few people are aware of it, bitamins cannot function, cannot be assimilated, without the aids of minerals. And though the body can synthesize some vitamins, it cannot manufacture a *single* mineral.

II

Vitamins: How and When

Where Vitamins Come From

Most vitamins are extracted from basic natural sources. Because vitamins are natural substances found in foods, the supplements you take — be they capsules, tablets, powders, or liquids — also come from foods. Though many of the vitamins can be synthesised, most are extracted from basic natural sources.

For example: Vitamin A usually comes from fish liver oil. Vitamin B complex comes from yeast or liver. Vitamin C is best when derived from rose hips, the berries found on the fruit of the rose after the petals have fallen off. And Vitamin E is generally extracted from soya beans, wheat germ, or corn.

Why Vitamins Come in Different Forms

Everyone's needs are different, and for this reason manufacturers have provided many vitamins in a variety of forms. Vitamins come in different forms because people do.

Tablets are the most common and convenient form. They're easier to store, carry, and have a longer shelf life than powders or liquids.

Capsules, like tablets, are convenient and easy to store, and are the usual supplement for oil-soluble vitamins such as A, D, and E.

Powders have advantages of extra potency [1 tsp. of many vitamin-C powders can give you as much as 4,000 mg.] and the added benefit of no fillers, binders, or additives for anyone with allergies.

Liquids are available for easy mixing with beverages and for people unable to swallow capsules and tablets.

Oil versus Dry or Water Soluble

The oil-soluble vitamins, such as A, D, E, and K are available and advisable in "dry" or water-soluble form for people who tend to get upset stomachs from oil, for acne sufferers, for anyone with a skin condition where oil ingestion is not advised, and for dieters who have cut most of the fat from their meals. [Fat-soluble vitamins need fat for proper assimilation. If you're on a low-fat diet and taking A, D, E or K supplements, I suggest you use the dry form.]

22

Synthetic versus Natural and Inorganic versus Organic

Synthetic vitamins can cause toxic reactions, while natural vitamins, even with high doses, don't. When I'm asked if there's a difference between synthetic and natural vitamins, I usually say only one — and that's to you. Though synthetic vitamins and minerals have produced satisfactory results, the benefits from natural vitamins, on a variety of levels, surpass them. Chemical analysis of both might appear the same, but there's more to natural vitamins because there's more to those substances in nature.

Synthetic vitamin C is just that, ascorbic acid and nothing more. Natural vitamin C from rose hips contains bioflavonoids, the entire C complex, which make the C much more effective.

Natural vitamin E, which can include all the tocopherols, just not alpha, is more potent than its synthetic double.

According to Dr. Theron G. Randolph, noted allergist: "A synthetically derived substance may cause a reaction in a chemically susceptible person when the same material of natural origin is tolerated, despite the two substances having identical chemical structures."

And as many who have tried both can attest, there are less gastrointestinal upsets with natural supplements. Also, and perhaps most important, synthetic vitamins can cause toxic reactions, while these reactions don't occur with natural vitamins when taken in higher than usual dosage.

The difference between inorganic and organic is not the same as the one between synthetic and natural, though that is the common misconception. All vitamins are organic. They are substances containing carbon.

Minerals, however, are inorganic. They do not contain carbon. But there are organic irons — ferrous gluconate, ferrous peptonate, and ferrous citrate. Ferrous sulphate, on the other hand, is an inorganic iron.

Chelation, and What It Means

First, pronounce it correctly. *Key' lation.* This is the process by which mineral substances are changed into their digestible form.

Common mineral supplements such as bonemeal and dolomite are often not chelated and must first be acted upon in the digestive process to form chelates before they are of use to the body. The natural chelating process is not performed efficiently in many people, and because of this a good deal of the mineral supplements they take are of little use.

When you realise that the body does not use whatever it takes in, that most of us do not digest our foods efficiently, that only 2 to 10 percent of inorganic iron taken into the body is actually absorbed, and, even with this small percentage, 50 per cent is then eliminated, you can recognise the importance of taking minerals that have been chelated. Chelated mineral supplements provide three to ten times greater assimilation than the nonchelated ones, and are well worth the small additional cost.

Time Release and Sustained Release

A major step forward in vitamin manufacturing has been the introduction of time release supplements. Time release also known as sustained release is a process by which vitamins are enrobed in micropellets [tiny time pills] and then combined into a special base for their release in a pattern that assures eight- to twelve-hour absorption. Most vitamins are water soluble and cannot be stored in the body. Without time release, they are quickly absorbed into the bloodstream, and, no matter how large the dose, are excreted in the urine within two or three hours.

Time-release supplements can offer optimum effectiveness, minimal excretary loss, and stable blood levels all during the day and through the night.

Fillers, Binders, Or What Else Are You Getting?

There's more to a vitamin supplement than meets the eye — and sometimes more than meets the label. Fillers, binders, lubricants, and the like do not have to be listed and often aren't. But if you'd like to know what you're swallowing, the following list should help.

Dilutents or fillers   These are inert materials added to the tablets to increase their bulk, in order to make them a practical size for compression. Dicalcium phosphate, which is an excellent source of calcium and phosphorus, is used in better brands. It is derived from purified mineral rocks. It is a white powder. Sorbitol and cellulose [plant fibre] are used occasionally.

Binders These substances give cohesive qualities to the powdered materials, otherwise the binders or granulators are the materials that hold the ingredients of the tablet together. Cellulose and ethyl cellulose are used most often. Cellulose is the main constituent of plant fibre. Other binders that can be used are:

acacia [gum arabic] — a vegetable gum

algin — alginic acid or sodium alginate — a plant carbohydrate derived from seaweed

lecithin and sorbitol are used occasionally

Lubricants A slick substance added to a tablet to keep it from sticking to the machines that punch it out. Calcium stearate and silica are commonly used. Calcium stearate is derived from natural vegetable oils. Silica is a natural white powder. Magnesium stearate can also be used.

Disintegrators Substances such as gum arabic, algin, and alginate are added to the tablet to facilitate its breakup or disintegration after ingestion.

Colours They make the tablet more aesthetic or elegant in appearance. Colours derived from natural sources, like chlorophyll, are best.

Flavours and sweeteners Used only in chewable tablets, the sweeteners are usually fructose [fruit sugar], malt dextrins, sorbitol, or maltose. Sucrose [sugar] is rarely used in better brands.

Coating materials These substances are used to protect the tablet from moisture. They also mask unpleasant flavour or odour and make the tablet easier to swallow. Zein is one of the substances. It is natural, derived from corn protein, and a clear film-coating agent. Brazil Wax, which is a natural product derived from palm trees, is also frequently used.

Drying agents These substances prevent water-absorbing [hygroscopic] materials from picking up moisture during processing, Silica gel is the most common drying agent.

Storage and Staying Power

Vitamin and mineral supplements should be stored in a cool dark place away from direct sunlight in a well-closed — preferably opaque — container. They do not have to be stored in the refrigerator unless you live in a desert climate. To guard against excessive moisture, place a few kernels of rice at the bottom of your vitamin bottle. The rice works as a natural absorbent.

If vitamins are kept cool and away from light, and remain well sealed, they should last for two to three years. Once a bottle is opened you can expect a twelve-month shelf life.

Our bodies tend to excrete in urine substances we take in on a four-hour basis, and this is particularly true of water-soluble vitamins such as B and C. On an empty stomach, B and C vitamins can leave the body as quickly as two hours after ingestion.

The oil-soluble vitamins, A, D, E and K, remain in the body for approximately twenty-hour hours, though excess amounts can be stored in the liver for much longer. Dry A and E do not stay in the body for long.

When and How to Take Supplements

The human body operates on a twenty-four hour cycle. Your cells do not go to sleep when you do, nor can they exist without continuous oxygen and nutrients. Therefore, for best results, space your supplements as evenly as possible during the day.

If you take your supplements all at once, do so after dinner, not breakfast. The prime time for taking supplements is after meals. Vitamins are organic substances and should be taken with other foods and minerals for best absorption. Because the water-soluble vitamins, especially B complex and C, are excreted fairly rapidly in the urine, a regimen of after breakfast, after lunch, and after dinner will provide you with the highest body level. If after each meal is not convenient, then half the amount should be taken after breakfast and the other half after dinner.

If you must take your vitamins all at once, then do so after the largest meal of the day. In other words, for best results, after dinner, not after breakfast, is the most desirable.

26

And remember, minerals are essential for proper vitamin absorption, so be sure to take your minerals and vitamins together.

What's Right for You

If you're unsure as to whether you'd be better off with a powder, a liquid, or a tablet, regular vitamin E or dry, taking supplements three times a day or time released, my advice to you is to experiment. If the supplement you're taking doesn't agree with you, try it in another form. Vitamin-C powder mixed in a beverage might be much easier to take than several large pills when you're coming down with a cold. If your face breaks out with vitamin E, try the dry form. Check Chapters IV to VI and the cautions in Chapter XXIII to make sure you know all you should about your supplement.

III

Vitamin-ese: a Glossary

Absorption: the process by which nutrients are passed into the bloodstream.

Acetate: a derivative of acetic acid.

Acetic acid: used as a synthetic flavouring agent, one of the first food additives (vinegar is approximately 4 to 6 percent acetic acid); it is found naturally in cheese, coffee, grapes, peaches, raspberries, and strawberries; Generally Recognized As Safe (GRAS) when used only in packaging.

Acetone: a colourless solvent for fat, oils, and waxes, which is obtained by fermentation (inhalation can irritate lungs, and large amounts have a narcotic effect).

Acid: a water-soluble substance with sour taste.

Adrenals: the glands, located above each kidney, that manufacture adrenaline.

Alkali: an acid-neutralizing substance (sodium bicarbonate is an alkali used for excess acidity in foods).

Allergen: a substance that causes an allergy.

Alzheimer's disease: a progressively degenerative disease, involved with loss of memory, which new research indicates might be helped with extra choline.

Amino acid chelates: chelated minerals that have been produced by many of the same processes nature uses to chelate minerals in the body; in the digestive tract, nature surrounds the elemental minerals with amino acid, permitting them to be absorbed into the bloodstream.

Amino acids: the organic compounds from which proteins are constructed; there are twenty-two known amino acids, but only nine are indispensable nutrients for man — histidine, isoleucine, leucine, lysine, total S-containing amino acids, total aromatic amino acids, threonine, tryptophan, and valine.

Anorexia: loss of appetite.

Antibiotic: any of various substances that are effective in inhibiting or destroying bacteria.

Anticoagulant: something that delays or prevents blood-clotting.

Antigen: any substance not normally present in the body that stimulates the body to produce antibodies.

Antihistamine: a drug used to reduce effects associated with histamine production in allergies and colds.

Antioxidant: a substance that can protect another substance from oxidation; added to foods to keep oxygen from changing the food's colour.

Antitoxin: an antibody formed in response to, and capable of neutralizing, a poison of biologic origin.

Assimilation: the process whereby nutrients are used by the body and changed into living tissue.

Ataxia: loss of coordinated movement caused by disease of nervous system.

ATP: a molecule called adrenosine triphosphate, the fuel of life, a nucleotide — building block of nucleic acid — that produces biological energy with B1, B2, B3, and pathothenic acid.

Avidin: a protein in egg white capable of inactivating biotin.

Bariatrician: a weight-control doctor.

B-Cells: white blood cells, made in the bone marrow, which produce antibodies upon instructions from T-cells, white blood cells manufactured in the thymus.

BHA: butylated hydroxyanisole; a preservative and antioxidant used in many products; insoluble in water; can be toxic to the kidneys.

BHT: butylated hydroxytoluene; a solid, white crystalline antioxidant used to retard spoilage of many foods; can be more toxic to the kidney than its nearly identical chemical cousin BHA.

Bioflavonoids: usually from orange and lemon rinds, these citrus-flavoured compounds needed to maintain healthy blood-vessel walls are widely available in plants, citrus fruits, and rose hips; known as vitamin P complex.

Calciferol: a colourless, odourless crystalline material, insoluble in water; soluble in fats; a synthetic form of vitamin D made by irradiating ergosterol with ultraviolet light.

Calcium gluconate: an organic form of calcium.

Capillary: a minute blood vessel, one of many that connect the arteries and veins.

Carcinogen: a cancer-causing substance.

Carotene: an orange-yellow pigment occurring in many plants and capable of being converted into vitamin A in the body.

Casein: the protein in milk that has become the standard by which protein quality is measured.

Catabolism: the metabolic change of nutrients or complex substances into simpler compounds, accompanied by a release of energy.

Catalyst: a substance that modifies, especially increases, the rate of chemical reaction without being consumed or changed in the process.

Chelation: a process by which mineral substances are changed into easily digestible form.

Chronic: of long duration; continuing; constant.

CNS: central nervous system.

Coenzyme: the major portion, though nonprotein, part of an enzyme; usually a B vitamin.

29

Collagen: the primary organic constituent of bone, cartilage, and connective tissue (becomes gelatin through boiling).

Congenital: condition existing at birth, not hereditary.

Dehydration: a condition resulting from an excessive loss of water from the body.

Dermatitis: an inflammation of the skin; a rash.

Desiccated: dried; preserved by removing moisture.

Dicalcium phosphate: a filler used in pills, which is derived from purified mineral rocks and is an excellent source of calcium and phosphorus.

Diluents: fillers; inert material added to tablets to increase their bulk in order to make them a practical size for compression.

Diuretic: tending to increase the flow of urine from the body.

DNA: deoxyribonucleic acid; the nucleic acid in chromosomes that is part of the chemical basis for hereditary characteristics.

Endogenous: being produced from within the body.

Enteric coated: a tablet coated so that it dissolves in the intestine, not in the stomach (which is acid).

Enuresis: bed-wetting.

Enzyme: a protein substance found in living cells that brings about chemical changes; necessary for digestion of food.

Excipient: any inert substance used as a dilutant or vehicle for a drug.

Exogenous: being derived or developed from external causes.

FDA: Food and Drug Administration.

Fibrin: an insoluble protein that forms the necessary fibrous network in the coagulation of blood.

Free-radicals: highly reactive chemical fragments that can produce an irritation of artery walls, start the arterio-sclerotic process if vitamin E is not present; generally harmful.

Fructose: a natural sugar occurring in fruits and honey; called fruit sugar; often used as a preservative for foodstuffs and an intravenous nutrient.

Galactosemia: a hereditary disorder in which milk becomes toxic as food.

Glucose: blood sugar; a product of the body's assimilation of carbohydrates and a major source of energy.

Glutamic acid: an amino acid present in all complete proteins;

usually manufactured from vegetable protein; used as a salt substitute and a flavour-intensifying agent.

Glutamine: an amino acid that constitutes, with glucose, the major nourishment used by the nervous system.

Gluten: a mixture of two proteins — gliadin and glutenin — present in wheat, rye, oats, and barley.

Glycogen: the body's chief storage carbohydrate, primarily in the liver.

GRAS: Generally Recognized As Safe; a list established by Congress to cover substances added to food.

Hesperidin: part of the C complex.

Holistic treatment: treatment of the whole person.

Homeostasis: the body's physiological equilibrium.

Hormone: a substance formed in endocrine organs and transported by body fluids to activate other specifically receptive organs.

Humectant: a substance that is used to preserve the moisture content of materials.

Hydrochloric acid: a normally acidic part of the body's gastric juice.

Hydrolyzed: put into water-soluble form.

Hydrolyzed protein chelate: water-soluble and chelated for easy assimilation.

Hypervitaminosis: a condition caused by an excessive ingestion of vitamins.

Hypoglycaemia: a condition caused by abnormally low blood sugar.

Hypovitaminosis: a deficiency disease owing to an absence of vitamins in the diet.

Ichthyosis: a condition characterized by a scaliness on the outer layer of skin.

Idiopathic: a condition whose causes are not yet known.

Immune: protected against disease.

Insulin: the hormone, secreted by the pancreas, concerned with the metabolism of sugar in the body.

IU: International Units.

Lactating: producing milk.

Laxative: a substance that stimulates evacuation of the bowels.

Linoleic acid: one of the polyunsaturated fats, a constituent of lecithin; known as vitamin F; indispensable for life, and must be obtained from foods.

Lipid: a fat or fatty substance.

Lipofuscin: age pigment in cells.

Lipotropic: preventing abnormal or excessive accumulation of fat in the liver.

Megavitamin therapy: treatment of illness with massive amounts of vitamins.

Metabolize: to undergo change by physical and chemical processes.

Mucopolysaccharide: thick gelatinous material that is found many places in the body; it glues cells together and lubricates joints.

Nitrites: used as fixatives in cured meats; can combine with natural stomach and food chemicals to cause dangerous cancer-causing agents called nitrosamines.

Orthomolecular: the right molecule used for the right treatment; doctors who practice preventive medicine and use vitamin therapies are known as orthomolecular physicians.

OSHA: Occupational Safety and Health Administration.

Oxalates: organic chemicals found in certain foods, especially spinach, which can combine with calcium to form calcium oxalate, an insoluble chemical the body cannot use.

PABA: para-aminobenzoic acid; a member of the B complex.

Palmitate: water-solublized vitamin A.

PKU (phenylketonuria): a hereditary disease caused by the lack of an enzyme needed to convert an essential amino acid (phenylalanine) into a form usable by the body; can cause mental retardation unless detected early.

Polyunsaturated fats: highly nonsaturated fats from vegetable sources; tend to lower blood cholesterol

Predigested protein: protein that has been processed for fast assimilation and can go directly to the bloodstream.

Provitamin: a vitamin precursor; a chemical substance necessary to produce a vitamin.

PUFA: polyunsaturated fatty acid.

RDA: Recommended Dietary Allowances as established by the Food and Nutrition Board, National Academy of Sciences, National Research Council.

RNA: the abbreviation used for ribonucleic acid.

Rose hips: a rich source of vitamin C; the nodule underneath the bud of a rose called a hip, in which the plant produces the vitamin C we extract.

Rutin: a substance extracted from buckwheat; part of the C complex.

Saturated fatty acids: usually solid at room temperature; higher proportions found in foods from animal sources; tend to raise blood cholesterol levels.

Sequestrant: a substance that absorbs ions and prevents changes that would affect flavour, texture, and colour of food; used for water softening.

Syncope: brief loss of consciousness; fainting.

Synergistic: the action of two or more substances to produce an effect that neither alone could accomplish.

Synthetic: produced artificially.

Systemic: capable of spreading through the entire body.

T-Cells: white blood cells, manufactured in the thymus, which protect the body from bacteria, viruses, and cancer-causing agents, while controlling the production of B-cells, which produce antibodies, and unwanted production of potentially harmful T-cells.

Teratological: monstrous or abnormal formations in animals or plants.

Tocopherols: the group of compounds (alpha, beta, delta, episilon, eta, gamma, and zeta) that make vitamin E; obtained through vacuum distillation of edible vegetable oils.

Toxicity: the quality or condition of being poisonous, harmful, or destructive.

Toxin: an organic poison produced in living or dead organisms.

Triglycerides: fatty substances in the blood.

Unsaturated fatty acids: most often liquid at room temperature; primarily found in vegetable fats.

USAN: United States Adopted Names Council; cosponsored by the American Pharmaceutical Association (APhA), the American Medical Association (AMA), and the United States Pharmacopia (USP) for the specific purpose of coining suitable, acceptable, nonproprietary names in the drug field.

USRDA: United States Recommended Daily Allowances.

Xerosis: a condition of dryness.
Zein: protein from corn.
Zyme: a fermenting substance.

IV

Everything You Always Wanted to Know About Vitamins But Had No One to Ask

Vitamin A

FACTS:

Vitamin A is fat soluble. It requires fats as well as minerals to be properly absorbed by your digestive tract.

It can be stored in your body and need not be replenished every day.

It occurs in two forms — preformed vitamin A, called retinol [found only in foods of animal origin], and provitamin A, known as carotene [provided by foods of both plant and animal origin].

Vitamin A is measured in USP Units [United States Pharmacopoeia], IU [International Units], and RE [Retinol Equivalents]. [See Chapter IX]

10,000 IU daily is the average adult dosage, though the need increases with greater body weight.

WHAT IT CAN DO FOR YOU:

Counteract night blindness, weak eyesight, and aid in the treatment of many eye disorders. [It permits formation of visual purple in the eye.]

Build resistance to respiratory infections.

Shorten the duration of diseases.

Keep the outer layers of your tissues and organs healthy.

Promote growth, strong bones, healthy skin, hair, teeth, and gums.

Help in the removal of age spots.

Help treat acne, impetigo, boils, carbuncles, and open ulcers when applied externally.

Aid in the treatment of emphysema and hyperthyroidism.

DEFICIENCY DISEASE:

Xerophthalmia, night blindness

BEST NATURAL SOURCES:

Fish liver oil, liver, carrots, green and yellow vegetables, eggs, milk and dairy products, margarine, and yellow fruits.

SUPPLEMENTS:

Usually available in two forms, one derived from natural fish liver oil and the other water dispersible. Water-dispersible supplements are either acetate or palmitate and recommended for anyone intolerant to oil, particularly acne sufferers.

Vitamin A acid [retin A] is sometimes prescribed for acne, but is available only by prescription. 10,000 to 25,000 IU are the most common daily doses.

TOXICITY:

More than 100,000 IU daily can produce toxic effects in adults, if taken for many months.

More than 18,500 IU daily can produce toxic effects in infants.

Toxicity symptoms include hair loss, nausea, vomiting, diarrhoea, scaly skin, blurred vision, rashes, bone pain, irregular menses, fatigue, headaches, and liver enlargement [See Chapter XXIII "Cautions".]

ENEMIES:

Polyunsaturated fatty acids with carotene work against vitamin A unless there are antioxidants present. [See Chapter XVI for antioxidants, and Chapter XVIII for drugs that deplete vitamins.]

PERSONAL ADVICE:

You need at least 10,000 IU vitamin A if you take more than 400 IU vitamin E daily.

If you are on the pill, your need for A is *decreased*.

If your weekly diet includes ample amounts of liver, carrots, spinach, sweet potatoes, or cantaloupe, it's unlikely you need an A supplement.

Vitamin A should *not* be taken with mineral oil.

Vitamin A works best with B complex, vitamin D, vitamin E, calcium, phosphorus, and zinc. (Zinc is what's needed by the liver to get vitamin A out of its storage deposits.)

Vitamin A also helps vitamin C from oxidizing.

If you are on a cholesterol-reducing drug such as *cholestyramine*, you'll have decreased vitamin A absorption and probably need a supplement.

Vitamin B$_1$ (Thiamine)

FACTS:

Water soluble. Like all the B-complex vitamins, any excess is excreted and not stored in the body. It must be replaced daily.

Measured in milligrams [mg.].

B vitamins are synergistic — they are more potent together than when used separately. B$_1$, B$_2$, and B$_6$ should be equally balanced [i.e. 50 mg. of B$_1$, 50 mg. of B$_2$, and 40 mg. of B$_6$] to work effectively.

The official RDA for adults is 1.2 to 1.4 mg. [During pregnancy and lactation 1.4 mg. is suggested.]

Need increases during illness, stress and surgery.

Known as the "morale vitamin" because of its beneficial effects on the nervous system and mental attitude.

Has a mild diuretic effect.

WHAT IT CAN DO FOR YOU:

Promote growth.

Aid digestion, especially of carbohydrates.
Improve your mental attitude.
Keep nervous system, muscles, and heart functioning normally.
Help fight air or seasickness
Relieve dental post-operative pain.
Aid in treatment of herpes zoster.

DEFICIENCY DISEASE:

Beriberi.

BEST NATURAL SOURCES:

Dried yeast, rice husks, whole wheat, oatmeal, peanuts, pork, most vegetables, bran, milk.

SUPPLEMENTS:

Available in low- and high-potency dosages — usually 50 mg. 100 mg., and 500 mg. It is most effective in B-complex formulas, balanced with B_2 and B_6. It is even more effective when the formula contains antistress pantothenic acid, folic acid, and B_{12}. 100 to 300 mg. are the most common daily doses.

TOXICITY:

No known toxicity for this water-soluble vitamin. Any excess is excreted in the urine and not stored to any degree in tissues or organs.

Rare excess symptoms include tremors, herpes, oedema, nervousness, rapid heartbeat, and allergies.

ENEMIES:

Cooking heat easily destroys this B vitamin. Other enemies of B_1 are caffeine, alcohol, food-processing methods, air, water, oestrogen, and sulphur drugs. [See Chapter XVIII for drugs that deplete vitamin.]

PERSONAL ADVICE:

If you are a smoker, drinker, or heavy sugar consumer, pregnant, nursing, or on the pill you have a greater need for this vitamin B_1.

If you are in the *habit* of taking an after-dinner anti-acid tablet you are losing the thiamine from your meal.

As with all stress conditions — disease, anxiety, trauma, post-surgery — your B-complex intake, which includes thiamine, should be increased.

Vitamin B$_2$ [**Riboflavin**]

FACTS:

Water soluble. Easily absorbed. The amount excreted depends on bodily needs and may be accompanied by protein loss. Like the other B vitamins it is not stored and must be replaced regularly through whole foods or supplements.

Also known as vitamin G.

Measured in milligrams [mg.]

Unlike thiamine, riboflavin is *not* destroyed by heat, oxidation, or acid.

For normal adults, 1.2 to 1.6 mg. is the RDA. Slightly higher amounts are suggested during pregnancy and lactation.

Increased need in stress situations.

America's most common vitamin deficiency is riboflavin.

WHAT IT CAN DO FOR YOU:

Aid in growth and reproduction.

Promote healthy skin, nails, hair.

Help eliminate sore mouth, lips, and tongue.

Benefit vision, alleviate eye fatigue.

Function with other substances to metabolise carbohydrates, fats, and proteins.

DEFICIENCY DISEASE:

Ariboflavinosis — mouth, lips, skin, genitalia lesions.

BEST NATURAL SOURCES:

Milk, liver, kidney, yeast, cheese, leafy green vegetables, fish, eggs.

SUPPLEMENTS:

Available in both low and high potencies — most commonly in 100 mg. doses. Like most of the B-complex vitamins, it is the most effective when in a well-balanced formula with the others. 100 to 300 mg. are the most common daily doses.

TOXICITY:

No known toxic effects.
Possible symptoms of minor excess including itching, numbness, sensations of burning or prickling.

ENEMIES:

Light — especially ultraviolet light — and alkalis are destructive to riboflavin [Opaque milk cartons now protect riboflavin that used to be destroyed in clear glass milk bottles.] Other natural enemies are water [B_2 dissolves in cooking liquids], sulphur drugs, oestrogen, alcohol. [See Chapter XVIII]

PERSONAL ADVICE:

If you are taking the pill, pregnant, or lactating, you need more vitamin B_2.
If you eat little red meat or dairy products you should increase your intake.
There is a strong likelihood of your being deficient in this vitamin if you are on a prolonged restricted diet for ulcers or diabetes. [In all cases where you are under medical treatment for a specific illness, check with your doctor before altering your present food regimen or embarking on a new one.]
All stress conditions require additional B complex.
If you are taking an anti-cancer drug such as *methotrexate* too much B_2 can cut down the drug's effectiveness.

Vitamin B₆[Pyridoxine]

FACTS:

Water soluble. Excreted within eight hours after ingestion

and, like the other B vitamins, needs to be replaced by whole food or supplements.

B_6 is actually a group of substances — pyridoxine, pyridoxinal, and pyridoxamine — that are closely related and function together.

Measured in milligrams [mg.].

Requirement increased when high-protein diets are consumed.

Must be present for the production of antibodies and red blood cells.

There is some evidence of synthesis by intestinal bacteria, and that a vegetable diet supplemented with cellulose is responsible.

The recommended adult intake is 1.6 to 2.0 mg. daily, with higher doses suggested during pregnancy and lactation.

Required for the proper absorption of vitamin B_{12}.

Necessary for the production of hydrochloric acid and magnesium.

WHAT IT CAN DO FOR YOU:

Properly assimilate protein and fat.

Aid in the conversion of tryptophan, an essential amino acid, to niacin.

Help prevent various nervous and skin disorders.

Alleviate nausea [many morning-sickness preparations that doctors prescribe include vitamin B_6].

Promote proper synthesis of antiaging nucleic acids.

Reduce night muscle spasms, leg cramps, hand numbness, certain forms of neuritis in the extremities.

Work as a natural diuretic.

DEFICIENCY DISEASE:
Anaemia, seborrhoeic dermatitis, glossitis.

BEST NATURAL SOURCES:

Brewer's yeast, wheat bran, wheat germ, liver, kidney, heart, cantaloupe, cabbage, blackstrap molasses, milk, eggs, beef.

SUPPLEMENTS:

Readily available in a wide range of dosages — from 50 to 500 mg. — in individual supplements as well as in B-complex and multivitamin formulas.

To prevent deficiencies in other B vitamins, pyridoxine should be taken in equal amounts with B_1 and B_2.

Can be purchased in time-disintegrating formulas that provide for gradual release up to ten hours.

TOXICITY:

Daily doses of 2–10 grams can cause neurological disorders.

Possible symptom of an oversupply of B_6 is night restlessness and too vivid dream recall.

Daily doses over 500 mg. are not recommended.

ENEMIES:

Long storage, canning, roasting or stewing of meat, water, food-processing techniques, alcohol, oestrogen. [See Chapter XVIII].

PERSONAL ADVICE:

If you are on the pill, you are more than likely to need increased amounts of B_6.

Heavy protein consumers need extra amounts of this vitamin.

Vitamin B_6 might decrease a diabetic's requirement for insulin, and if the dosage is not adjusted, a low-blood-sugar reaction could result.

Arthritis sufferers being treated with *penicillamine* should be taking supplements of this vitamin.

This vitamin works best with vitamin B_1, vitamin B_2, pantothenic acid, vitamin C, and magnesium.

Supplements for this vitamin should *not* be taken by anyone under *levodopa* treatment for Parkinson's disease! (Ask your doctor about a drug which can bypass this particular adverse vitamin interaction.)

Vitamin B_{12}[Cobalamin]

FACTS: Water soluble and effective in very small doses.

Commonly known as the "red vitamin", also cyanocobalamin.

Measured in micrograms [mcg.].

The only vitamin that contains essential mineral elements.

Not well assimilated through the stomach. Needs to be combined with calcium during absorption to benefit body properly.

Recommended adult dose is 3 mcg., with larger amounts suggested for pregnant and lactating women.

A diet low in B_1 and high in folic acid [such as a vegetarian diet] often hides a vitamin-B_{12} deficiency.

A properly functioning thyroid gland helps B_{12} absorption. Symptoms of B_{12} deficiency may take more than five years to appear after body stores have been depleted.

WHAT IT CAN DO FOR YOU:

Form and regenerate red blood cells, thereby preventing anaemia.

Promote growth and increase appetite in children.

Increase energy.

Maintain a healthy nervous system.

Properly utilise fats, carbohydrates, and protein.

Relieve irritability.

Improve concentration, memory, and balance.

DEFICIENCY DISEASE:

Pernicious anaemia, brain damage.

BEST NATURAL SOURCES:

Liver, beef, pork, eggs, milk, cheese, kidney.

SUPPLEMENTS:

Because B_{12} is not absorbed well through the stomach, I recommend the time-release form of tablet so that it can be assimilated in the small intestine.

Supplements are available in a variety of strengths from 50 mcg. to 2,000 mcg.

Doctors routinely give vitamin-B_{12} injections. If there is a severe indication of deficiency or extreme fatigue, this method might be the supplementation that is called for.

Daily doses most often used are 5 to 100 mcg.

There have been no cases reported ov vitamin-B_{12} toxicity, even on megadose regimens.

Enemies:

Acids and alkalis, water, sunlight, alcohol, oestrogen, sleeping pills. [See Chapter XVIII.]

Personal Advice:

If you are a vegetarian and have excluded eggs and dairy products from your diet, then you need B_{12} supplementation.

Combined with folic acid, B_{12} can be a most effective revitaliser.

Surprisingly, heavy protein consumers may also need extra amounts of this vitamin, which works synergistically with almost all other B vitamins as well as vitamins A, E, and C.

Women may find B_{12} helpful — as part of a B complex — during and just prior to menstruation.

Vitamin B_{13} [Orotic Acid]

Facts:

Metabolises folic acid and vitamin B_{12}.
No RDA has been established.

What It Can Do For You:

Possibly prevent certain liver problems and premature aging.
Aid in the treatment of multiple sclerosis.

Deficiency Disease:

Deficiency symptoms and diseases related to this vitamin are still uncertain.

Best Natural Sources:

Root vegetables, whey, the liquid portion of soured or curdled milk.

SUPPLEMENTS:

Available as calcium orotate in supplemental form.

TOXICITY:

Too little is known at this time to establish guidelines.

ENEMIES:

Water and sunlight.

PERSONAL ADVICE:

Unfortunately not enough research has been done on this vitamin for recommendations to be made.

Vitamin B$_{15}$[Pangamic Acid]

FACTS:

Water soluble.
Because its essential requirement for diet has not been proved, it is not a vitamin in the strict sense.
Measured in milligrams [mg.].
Works much like vitamin E in that it is an antioxidant.
Introduced and approved by the Russians while the U.S. Food and Drug Administration has doubts about it.
Action is often improved by being taken with Vitamins A and E.

WHAT IT CAN DO FOR YOU:*

Extend cell life span.
Neutralise the craving for liquor.
Speed recovery from fatigue.
Lower blood cholesterol levels.
Protect against pollutants.
Aid in protein synthesis.
Relieve symptoms of angina and asthma.
Protect the liver against cirrhosis.

---

* U.S. research in the case of B$_{15}$ has been limited. The list of benefits given here is based on my study of Soviet tests.

Ward off hangovers.
Stimulate immunity responses.

DEFICIENCY DISEASE:

Again, research has been limited, but indications point to glandular and nerve disorders, heart disease, and diminished oxygenation of living tissue.

BEST NATURAL SOURCES:

Brewer's yeast, whole brown rice, whole grains, pumpkin seeds, sesame seeds.

SUPPLEMENTS:

Usually available in 50-mg. strengths.
Daily doses most often used are 50 to 150 mgs.

TOXICITY:

There have been no reported cases of toxicity. Some people say they have experienced nausea on beginning a B_{15} regimen, but this usually disappears after a few days and can be alleviated by taking the B_{15} supplement after the day's largest meal.

ENEMIES:

Water and sunlight.

PERSONAL ADVICE:

Despite the controversy, I have found B_{15} effective and believe most diets would benefit from supplementation.

If you are an athlete or just want to feel like one, I suggest one 50-mg. tablet in the morning with breakfast and one in the evening with dinner.

An important supplement for residents of big cities and high-density pollution areas.

Vitamin B_{17} [Laetrile]

FACTS:

One of the most controversial "vitamins" of the decade.

Chemically a compound of two sugar molecules [one benzaldehyde and one cyanide] called an amygdalin.

Known as nitrilosides when used in medical doses.

Obtained from apricot pits.

One B vitamin that is not present in brewer's yeast.

Touted as a cancer treatment in most of the United States at this date and legal in fifteen states but rejected by the Food and Drug Administration on the grounds that it might be poisonous due to its cyanide content.

WHAT IT CAN DO FOR YOU:

It is *purported* to have specific cancer-controlling and preventative properties.

DEFICIENCY DISEASE:

May lead to diminished resistance to cancer.

BEST NATURAL SOURCES:

A small amount of laetrile is found in the whole kernels of apricots, apples, cherries, peaches, plums, and nectarines.

SUPPLEMENTS:

Daily doses most often used are .25 to 1.0 g.

TOXICITY:

Though no toxicity levels have been established yet, taking excessive amounts of laetrile could be dangerous. Cumulative amounts of more than 3.0 g. can be ingested safely, but not more than 1.0 g. at any one time.

According to the *Nutrition Almanac*, five to thirty apricot kernels eaten through the day, but never all at the same time, can be a sufficient preventive amount.

PERSONAL ADVICE:

There is now extensive literature available on laetrile. I strongly advise personal research and a consultation with a physician before embarking on any regimen involving B_{17}.

Biotin [Coenzyme R or Vitamin H]

FACTS:

Water soluble, and another fairly recent member of the B-complex family.

Usually measured in micrograms [mcg.].

Synthesis of ascorbic acid requires biotin.

Essential for normal metabolism of fat and protein.

The RDA for adults is 150 to 300 mcg.

Can be synthesised by intestinal bacteria.

Raw eggs prevent absorption by the body.

Synergistic with B_2, B_6, niacin, A, and in maintaining healthy skin.

WHAT IT CAN DO FOR YOU:

Aid in keeping hair from turning grey.

Help in preventive treatment for baldness.

Ease muscle pains.

Alleviate eczema and dermatitis.

DEFICIENCY DISEASE:

Eczema of face and body, extreme exhaustion, impairment of fat metabolism.

BEST NATURAL SOURCES:

Nuts, fruits, brewer's yeast, beef liver, egg yolk, milk, kidney, and unpolished rice.

SUPPLEMENTS:

Biotin is usually included in most B-complex supplements and multiple-vitamin tablets.

Daily doses most often used are 25 to 300 mcg.

TOXICITY:

There are no known cases of biotin toxicity.

ENEMIES:

Raw egg white [which contains avidin, a protein that prevents biotin absorption], water, sulphur drugs, oestrogen, food-processing techniques, and alcohol. [See Chapter XVIII].

PERSONAL ADVICE:

If you drink a lot of eggnogs made with raw eggs you probably need biotin supplementation.

Be sure you're getting at least 25 mcg. daily if you are on antibiotics or sulfa drugs.

Balding men might find that a biotin supplement *may* keep their hair there longer.

Keep in mind that biotin works synergistically — and more effectively — with B_2, B_6, niacin and A.

Vitamin C[Ascorbic Acid, Cevitamin Acid]

FACTS:

Water soluble.

Most animals synthesise their own vitamin C, but man, apes, and guinea pigs must rely upon dietary sources.

Plays a primary role in the formation of collagen, which is important for the growth and repair of body tissue cells, gums, blood vessels, bones, and teeth.

Helps in the body's absorption of iron.

Measured in milligrams [mg.].

Used up more rapidly under stress conditions.

The RDA for adults in 45 mg. [higher doses recommended during pregnancy and lactation].

Recommended as a preventive for crib death or sudden infant death syndrome [SIDS].

Smokers and older persons have greater need for vitamin C. [Each cigarette destroys 25 mg.]

WHAT IT CAN DO FOR YOU:

Heal wounds, burns, and bleeding gums.

Accelerate healing after surgery.

Help in decreasing blood cholesterol.

Aid in preventing many types of viral and bacterial infections.

Act as a natural laxative.

Lower incidence of blood clots in veins.

Aid in treatment and prevention of the common cold.

Extend life by enabling protein cells to hold together.
Reduce effects of many allergy-producing substances.
Prevent scurvy.

Decrease infections by 25 percent and cancers by 75 percent if taken in 1,000-mg. to 10,000-mg. daily dosage, according to Dr. Linus Pauling.

DEFICIENCY DISEASE:

Scurvy.

BEST NATURAL SOURCES:

Citrus fruits, berries, green and leafy vegetables, tomatoes, cauliflower, potatoes and sweet potatoes.

SUPPLEMENTS:

Vitamin C is one of the most widely taken supplements. It is available in conventional pills and effervescent tablets, time-release tablets, syrups, powders and pastilles.

The form that is *pure* vitamin C is derived from corn dextrose [though no corn or dextrose remains.]

The difference between "natural" or "organic" vitamin C and ordinary ascorbic acid is primarily in the individual's ability to digest it.

The best vitamin-C supplement is one that contains the complete C complex of bioflavonoids, hesperidin, and rutin. [Sometimes these are labelled citrus salts.]

Tablets and capsules are usually supplied in strengths up to 1,000 mg. and in powder form sometimes 5,000 mg. per tsp.

Daily doses most often used are 500 mg. to 4 g.

Rose hips vitamin C contains bioflavonoids and other enzymes that help C assimilate. They are the richest natural sources of vitamin C. [The C is actually manufactured under the bud of the rose — called a hip.]

TOXICITY:

No proven toxic effects, though excessive intake might cause some unpleasant side effects in specific cases. Occasional diarrhoea, excess urination, kidney stones, and skin rashes may develop on megadoses. Cut back dosage if any of these occurs.

Vitamin C should not be used by cancer patients undergoing radiation or chemotherapy.

ENEMIES:

Water, cooking, heat, light, oxygen, smoking. [See Chapter XVIII]

PERSONAL ADVICE:

Because vitamin C is excreted in two to three hours, depending on the quality of food in the stomach, and it is important to maintain a constant high level of C in the bloodstream at all times, I recommend a time-release tablet for optimum effectiveness.

Large doses of vitamin C can alter the results of laboratory tests. If you're going to have any blood or urine testing, be sure to inform your doctor that you're taking vitamin C so that no errors will be made in diagnosis. (Vitamin C can mask the presence of blood in stool.)

Diabetics should be aware that testing the urine for sugar could be inaccurate if you're taking a lot of vitamin C. (But there are testing kits available that aren't affected by vitamin C. Ask your pharmacist or physician.)

To maximize the effectiveness of vitamin C, remember that it works best in conjunction with bioflavonoids, calcium, and magnesium.

If you're taking over 750 mg. daily, I suggest a magnesium supplement. This is an effective deterrent against kidney stones.

Carbon monoxide destroys vitamin C, so city dwellers should definitely up their intake.

You need extra C if you are on the pill.

I recommend increasing C doses if you take aspirin or simply want your other vitamins to work better.

If you take ginseng, it's better to take it three hours before or after taking vitamin C or foods high in the vitamin.

Calcium Pantothenate [Pantothenic Acid, Panthenol, Vitamin B_5]

FACTS:

Water soluble, another member of the B-complex family.
Helps in cell building, maintaining normal growth, and development of the central nervous system.
Vital for the proper functioning of the adrenal glands.
Essential for conversion of fat and sugar to energy.
Necessary for synthesis of antibodies, for utilisation of PABA and choline.
The RDA [as set by the FDA] is 10 mg. for adults.
Can be synthesised in the body by intestinal bacteria.

WHAT IT CAN DO FOR YOU:

Aid in wound healing.
Fight infection by building antibodies.
Treat post-operative shock.
Prevent fatigue.
Reduce adverse and toxic effects of many antibiotics.

DEFICIENCY DISEASE:

Hypoglycaemia, duodenal ulcers, blood and skin disorders.

BEST NATURAL SOURCES:

Meat, whole grains, wheat germ, bran, kidney, liver, heart, green vegetables, brewer's yeast, nuts, chicken, crude molasses.

SUPPLEMENTS:

Most commonly found in B-complex formulas in a variety of strengths from 10 to 100 mg.
10 to 300 mg. are the daily doses usually taken.

TOXICITY:

No known toxic effects.

ENEMIES:

Heat, food-processing techniques, canning, caffeine, sulphur drugs, sleeping pills, oestrogen, alcohol. [See Chapter XVIII.]

If you frequently have tingling hands and feet, you might try increasing your pantothenic acid intake — in combination with other B vitamins.

Pantothenic acid can help provide a defence against a stress situation that you foresee or in which you are involved.

1,000 mg. daily has been found effective in reducing the pain of arthritis, in some cases. If you suffer from allergies relief could be just a B_5 and C away. Try taking 1,000 mg. of each – with food – morning and evening.

Choline

Facts:

A member of the B-complex family and a lipotropic [Fat emulsifier].

Works with inositol [another B-complex member] to utilise fats and cholesterol.

One of the few substances able to penetrate the so-called blood-brain barrier, which ordinarily protects the brain against variations in the daily diet, and go directly into the brain cells to produce a chemical that aids memory.

The RDA has not yet been established, though it's estimated that the average adult diet contains between 500 and 900 mg. a day.

Seems to emulsify cholesterol so that it doesn't settle on artery walls or in the gallbladder.

What It Can Do For You:

Help control cholesterol build up.

Aid in the sending of nerve impulses, specifically those in the brain used in the formation of memory.

Assist in conquering the problem of memory loss in later years.

Help eliminate poisons and drugs from your system by aiding the liver.

Produce a soothing effect.

Aids in the treatment of Alzheimer's disease.

DEFICIENCY DISEASE:

May result in cirrhosis and fatty degeneration of liver, hardening of the arteries, and possibly Alzheimer's disease.

BEST NATURAL SOURCES:

Egg yolks, brain, heart, green leafy vegetables, yeast, liver, wheat germ, and, in small amounts, in lecithin.

SUPPLEMENTS:

Six lecithin capsules, made from soya beans, contain 244 mg. each of inositol and choline.

The average B-complex supplement contains approximately 50 mg. of choline and inositol.

Daily doses most often used are 500 to 1,000 mg.

TOXICITY:

None known.

ENEMIES:

Water, sulfa drugs, oestrogen, food processing, and alcohol. [See Chapter XVIII.]

PERSONAL ADVICE:

Always take choline with your other B vitamins.

If you are often nervous or "twitchy" it might help to increase your choline.

If you are taking lecithin, you probably need a chelated calcium supplement to keep your phosphorus and calcium in balance, since choline seems to increase the body's phosphorus.

Try getting more choline into your diet as a way to a better memory.

Vitamin D [Calciferol, Viosterol, Ergosterol, "Sunshine Vitamin"]

FACTS:

Fat soluble. Acquired through sunlight or diet. [Ultraviolet sunrays act on the oils of the skin to produce the vitamin, which is then absorbed into the body.]

When taken orally, vitamin D is absorbed with fats through the intestinal walls.

Measured in International Units [IU].

The RDA for adults is 400 IU or 5–10 mcg.

Smog reduces the vitamin-D-producing sunshine rays.

After a suntan is established, vitamin-D production through the skin stops.

WHAT IT CAN DO FOR YOU:

Properly utilise calcium and phosphorus necessary for strong bones and teeth.

Taken with vitamins A and C it can aid in preventing colds.

Help in treatment of conjunctivitis.

Aids in assimilating vitamin A.

DEFICIENCY DISEASE:

Rickets, severe tooth decay, osteomalacia, senile osteoporosis.

BEST NATURAL SOURCES:

Fish liver oils, sardines, herring, salmon, tuna, milk and dairy products.

SUPPLEMENTS:

Usually supplied in 400 IU capsules, the vitamin itself is derived from fish liver oil.

Daily doses most often taken are 400 to 1,000 IU.

TOXICITY:

25,000 IU daily over an extended period of time can produce toxic effects in adults.

Dosages of over 5,000 IU daily might affect some individuals adversely.

Signs of toxicity are unusual thirst, sore eyes, itching skin, vomiting, diarrhoea, urinary urgency, abnormal calcium deposits in blood-vessel walls, liver, lungs, kidney and stomach.

Mineral oil, smog. [See Chapter XVIII]

PERSONAL ADVICE:

City dwellers, especially those in areas of high smog density, should increase their vitamin-D intake.

Night workers, nuns, and others whose clothing of life-style keeps them from sunlight should increase the D in their diet.

Children who don't drink D-fortified milk should increase their intake of D.

Dark-skinned people living in northern climates usually need an increase in vitamin D.

Vitamin E [Tocopherol]

FACTS:

Fat soluble and stored in the liver, fatty tissues, heart, muscles, testes, uterus, blood, adrenal and pituitary glands.

Formerly measured by weight, but now generally designated according to its biological activity in International Units [IU]. With this vitamin 1 IU is the same as 1 mg.

Composed of compounds called tocopherols. One of the eight tocopherols — alpha, beta, gamma, delta, epsilon, zeta, eta, and theta — alphatocopherol is the most effective.

An active antioxidant, prevents oxidation of fat compounds as well as that of vitamin A, selenium, two sulphur amino acids, and some vitamin C.

Enhances activity of vitamin A.

The RDA for adults is 12 IU to 15 IU. [This requirement is based on the National Research Council's 1974 revised allowances. The U.S. RDA for adults is 30 IU.]

60 to 70 percent of daily doses are excreted in faeces. Unlike other fat-soluble vitamins, E is stored in the body for a relatively short time, much like B and C.

Important as a vasodilator and an anticoagulant.

Products with 25 mcg. of selenium for each 200 units of E increase E's potency.

WHAT IT CAN DO FOR YOU:

Keeping you looking younger by retarding cellular aging due to oxidation.

Supply oxygen to the body to give you more endurance.

Protect your lungs against air pollution by working with vitamin A.

Prevent and dissolve blood clots.

Alleviate fatigue.

Prevent thick scar formation externally [when applied topically — it can be absorbed through the skin] and internally.

Accelerate healing of burns.

Working as a diuretic, it can lower blood pressure.

Aid in prevention of miscarriages.

DEFICIENCY DISEASE:

Destruction of red blood cells, muscle degeneration, some anaemias and reproductive disorders.

BEST NATURAL SOURCES:

Wheat germ, soya beans, vegetable oils, broccoli, Brussels sprouts, leafy greens, spinach, enriched flour, whole wheat, whole-grain cereals, and eggs.

SUPPLEMENTS:

Available in oil-base capsules as well as water-soluble dry-base tablets.

Usually supplied in strengths from 100 to 1,000 IU. The dry form is recommended for anyone who cannot tolerate oil or whose skin condition is aggravated by oil.

Daily doses most often used are 200 to 2,000 IU.

TOXICITY:

Essentially nontoxic.

ENEMIES:

Heat, oxygen, freezing temperatures, food processing, iron, chlorine, mineral oil. [See Chapter XVIII.]

If you're on a diet high in polyunsaturated oils, you might need additional vitamin E.

Inorganic iron [ferrous sulphate] destroys vitamin E, so the two should not be taken together. If you're using a supplement containing any ferrous sulphate, E should be taken at least eight hours before or after.

Ferrous gluconate, peptonate, citrate, or fumerate [organic iron complexes] do not destroy E.

If you have chlorinated drinking water, you need more vitamin E.

Pregnant or lactating women, as well as those on the pill or taking hormones, need increased vitamin E.

I advise women going through menopause to increase their E intake. (Mixed tocopherols are recommended 400 to 1,200 IU daily.)

Vitamin F [Unsaturated Fatty Acids — Linoleic, Linolenic and Arachidonic]

Facts:

Fat soluble, made up of unsaturated fatty acids obtained from foods.

Measured in milligrams [mg.].

No RDA has been established, but the National Research Council has suggested that at least 1 percent of total calories should include essential unsaturated fatty acids.

Unsaturated fat helps burn saturated fat, with intake balanced two to one.

Twelve teaspoons sunflower seeds or eighteen pecan halves can furnish a day's complete supply.

If there is sufficient linoleic acid, the other two fatty acids can be synthesised.

Heavy carbohydrate consumption increases need.

What It Can Do For You:

Aid in preventing cholesterol deposits in the arteries.
Promote healthy skin and hair.

Give some degree of protection against the harmful effects of X-rays.

Aid in growth and well-being by influencing glandular activity and making calcium available to cells.

Combat heart disease.

Aid in weight reduction by burning saturated fats.

DEFICIENCY DISEASE:

Eczema, acne.

BEST NATURAL SOURCES:

Vegetable oils — wheat germ, linseed, sunflower, safflower, soyabean, and peanut — peanuts, sunflower seeds, walnuts, pecans, almonds, avocados.

SUPPLEMENTS:

Comes in capsules of 100- to 150-mg. strengths.

TOXICITY:

No known toxic effects, but an excess can lead to unwanted pounds.

ENEMIES:

Saturated fats, heat, oxygen.

PERSONAL ADVICE:

For best absorption of vitamin F, take vitamin E with it at mealtimes.

If you are a heavy carbohydrate consumer, you need more vitamin F.

Anyone worried about cholesterol build up should be getting the proper intake of F.

Though most nuts are fine sources of unsaturated fatty acids, Brazil nuts and cashews are *not*

Watch out for fad diets high in saturated fats.

Folic Acid [Folacin]

FACTS:

Water soluble, another member of the B complex.
Measured in micrograms [mcg.].
Essential to the formation of red blood cells.
Aid in protein metabolism.
The official Recommended Daily Dietary Allowance for adults is 400 mcg., and twice the amount for pregnant and lactating women.
Important for the production of nucleic acids [RNA and DNA].
Essential for division of body cells.
Needed for utilisation of sugar and amino acids.
Can be destroyed by being stored, unprotected, at room temperature for extended time periods.

WHAT IT CAN DO FOR YOU:

Improve lactation.
Protect against intestinal parasites and food poisoning.
Promote healthier-looking skin.
Act as an analgesic for pain.
May delay hair greying when used in conjunction with pantothenic acid and PABA.
Increase appetite, if you are debilitated [run down].
Act as a preventive for canker sores.
Help ward off anaemia.

DEFICIENCY DISEASE:

Nutritional macrocytic anaemia.

BEST NATURAL SOURCES:

Deep-green leafy vegetables, carrots, tortula yeast, liver, egg yolk, melon, apricots, pumpkins, avocados, beans, whole wheat and dark rye flour.

SUPPLEMENTS:

Usually supplied in 400-mcg. and 800-mcg. strengths. Strengths of 1 mg. [1,000 mcg.] are available by prescription only.

59

400 mcg. are sometimes supplied in B-complex formulas, but often only 100 mcg. [Check labels.]

Daily doses most often used are 400 mcg. to 5 mg.

TOXICITY:

No known toxic effects, though a few people experience allergic skin reactions.

ENEMIES:

Water, sulfa drugs, sunlight, oestrogen, food processing [especially boiling], heat. [See Chapter XVIII.]

PERSONAL ADVICE:

If you are a heavy drinker, it is advisable to increase your folic-acid intake.

High vitamin-C intake increases excretion of folic acid, and anyone taking more than 2 g. of C should probably up his folic acid.

If you are on Dilantin or take oestrogens, sulphonamides, phenobarbital, or aspirin, I suggest increasing folic acid.

I've found that many people taking 1 to 5 mg. daily, for a short period of time, have reversed several types of skin discolouration. If this is a problem to you, it's worth checking out a nutritionally orientated doctor about the possibility.

If you are getting sick, or fighting an illness, make sure your stress supplement has ample folic acid. When folic acid is deficient, so are your antibodies.

Inositol

FACTS:

Water soluble, another member of the B complex, and a lipotropic.

Measured in milligrams [mg.].

Combines with choline to form lecithin.

Metabolises fats and cholesterol.

Daily dietary allowances have not yet been established, but the average healthy adult get approximately 1 g. a day.

Like choline, it has been found important in nourishing brain cells.

WHAT IT CAN DO FOR YOU:

Help lower cholesterol levels.
Promote healthy hair — aid in preventing fall-out.
Help in preventing eczema.
Aid in redistribution of body fat.

DEFICIENCY DISEASE:

Eczema.

BEST NATURAL SOURCES:

Liver, brewer's yeast, dried lima beans, beef brains and heart, cantaloupe, grapefruit, raisins, wheat germ, unrefined molasses, peanuts, cabbage.

SUPPLEMENTS:

As with choline, six soy bean-based lecithin capsules contain approximately 244 mg. each of inositol and choline.
Available in lecithin powders that mix well with liquids. Most B-complex supplements contain approximately 100 mg. of choline and inositol.
Daily doses most often used are 250 to 500 mg.

TOXICITY:

No known toxic effects.

ENEMIES:

Water, sulfa drugs, oestrogen, food processing, alcohol, and coffee. [See Chapter XVIII.]

PERSONAL ADVICE:

Take inositol with choline and your other B vitamins.
If you are a heavy coffee drinker, you probably need supplemental inositol.
If you take lecithin, I advise a supplement of chelated calcium to keep your phosphorus and calcium in balance, as both inositol and choline seem to raise phosphorus levels.

A good way to maximise the effectiveness of your vitamin E is to get enough inositol and choline.

Vitamin K [Menadione]

FACTS:

Fat soluble.
Usually measured in micrograms [mcg.].
There is a trio of K vitamins, K_1 and K_2 can be formed by natural bacteria in the intestines. K_3 is a synthetic.
No dietary allowance has yet been established, but an adult intake of approximately 300 mcg. is generally considered adequate. Newborn infants need more.
Essential in the formation of prothrombin, a blood-clotting chemical.

WHAT IT CAN DO FOR YOU:

Help in preventing internal bleeding and haemorrhages.
Aid in reducing excessive menstrual flow.
Promote proper blood clotting.

DEFICIENCY DISEASE:

Coeliac disease, sprue, colitis.

BEST NATURAL SOURCES:

Yoghurt, alfalfa, egg yolk, safflower oil, soyabean oil, fish liver oils, kelp, leafy green vegetables.

SUPPLEMENTS:

The abundance of natural vitamin K generally makes supplementation unnecessary.
It is not included ordinarily in multiple-vitamin capsules.

TOXICITY:

More than 500 mcg. of synthetic vitamin K is not recommended.

ENEMIES:

X-rays and radiation, frozen foods, aspirin, air pollution, mineral oil. [See Chapter XVIII.]

PERSONAL ADVICE:

Excessive diarrhoea can be a symptom of vitamin K deficiency, but before self-supplementing, see a doctor.

Yoghurt is your best defence against a vitamin K deficiency.

If you have nosebleeds often, try increasing your K through natural food sources. Alfalfa tablets might help. If you are taking an anticoagulant be aware that this vitamin (even in natural foods) can reverse the drug's effects.

Niacin [Nicotinic Acid, Niacinamide, Nicotinamide]

FACTS:

Water soluble and a member of the B-complex family, known as B_3.

Usually measured in milligrams [mg].

Using the amino acid tryptophan, the body can manufacture its own niacin.

A person whose body is deficient in B_1, B_2, and B_6 will not be able to produce niacin from tryptophan.

lack of niacin can bring about negative personality changes.

The RDA, according to the National Research Council, is 12 to 18 mg. for adults.

Essential for synthesis of sex hormones [oestrogen, progesterone, testosterone], as well as cortisone, thyroxin, and insulin.

Necessary for healthy nervous system and brain function.

Niacinamide is more generally used since it minimises the flushing and itching of the skin that frequently occurs with the nicotinic acid form of niacin. [The flush, by the way, is not serious and usually disappears in about twenty minutes. Drinking a glass of water helps.]

WHAT IT CAN DO FOR YOU:

Aid in promoting a healthy digestive system, alleviate gastrointestinal disturbances.

Give you healthier-looking skin.
Help prevent and ease severity of migraine headaches.
Increase circulation and reduce high blood pressure.
East some attacks of diarrhoea.
Reduce the unpleasant symptoms of vertigo in Ménière's syndrome.
Increase energy through proper utilisation of food.
Help eliminate canker sores and, often, bad breath.
Reduce cholesterol.

DEFICIENCY DISEASE:

Pellagra.

BEST NATURAL SOURCES:

Liver, lean meat, whole wheat products, brewers's yeast, kidney, wheat germ, fish, eggs, roasted peanuts, the white meat of poultry, avocados, dates, figs, prunes.

SUPPLEMENTS:

Available as niacin and niacinamide. [The only difference is that niacin — nicotinic acid — might cause flushing and niacinamide — nicotinamide — will not. If you prefer niacin, you can minimise the flushing by taking your pill on a full stomach or with an equivalent amount of inositol.]

Usually found in 50 to 1,000-mg. doses in pill and powder form.

50 to 100 mg. are ordinarily included in the better B-complex formulas and multivitamin preparations. [Check labels.]

TOXICITY:

Essentially nontoxic, except for side effects resulting from doses above 100 mg.

Some sensitive individuals might experience burning or itching skin.

ENEMIES:

Water, sulfa drugs, alcohol, food-processing techniques, sleeping pills, oestrogen. [See Chapter XVIII.]

PERSONAL ADVICE:

If you're taking antibiotics and suddenly find your niacin flushes becoming severe, don't be alarmed.

I's quite common. You'll probably be more comfortable if you switch to niacinamide.

If you have a cholesterol problem, increasing your niacin intake can help.

Skin that is particularly sensitive to sunlight is often an early indicator of niacin deficiency.

Do not give your pets large doses of niacin. It can cause flushing and sweating, greatly distressing the animal and you.

Vitamin P [C Complex, Citrus Bioflavonoids, Rutin, Hesperidin]

FACTS:

Water soluble and composed of citrin, rutin, and hesperidin, as well as flavones and flavonals.

Usually measured in milligrams [mg.].

Necessary for the proper function and absorption of vitamin C.

Flavonoids are the substances that provide that yellow and orange colour in citrus foods.

Also called the capillary permeability factor. [P stands for permeability.] The prime function of bioflavonoids is to increase capillary strength and regulate absorption.

Aids vitamin C in keeping connective tissues healthy.

No daily allowance has been established, but most nutritionists agree that for every 500 mg. of vitamin C you should have at least 100 mg. of bioflavonoids.

Works synergistically with vitamin C.

WHAT IT CAN DO FOR YOU:

Prevent vitamin C from being destroyed by oxidation.

Strengthen the walls of capillaries, thereby preventing bruising.

Help build resistance to infection.

Aid in preventing and healing bleeding gums.

Increase the effectiveness of vitamin C.

Help in the treatment of edema and dizziness due to disease of the inner ear.

DEFICIENCY DISEASE:

Capillary fragility.

BEST NATURAL SOURCES:

The white skin and segment part of citrus fruit — lemons, oranges, grapefruit. Also in apricots, buckwheat, blackberries, cherries and rose hips.

SUPPLEMENTS:

Available usually in a C complex or by itself. Most often there are 500 mg. of bioflavonoids to 50 mg. of rutin and hesperidin. [If the ratio of rutin and hesperidin is not equal, it should be twice as much rutin.]

All C supplements work better with bioflavonoids.

Most common doses of rutin and hesperidin are 100 mg. three times a day.

TOXICITY:

No known toxicity.

ENEMIES:

Water, cooking, heat, light, oxygen, smoking.

PERSONAL ADVICE:

Menopausal women can usually find some effective relief from hot flushes with an increase in bioflavonoids taken in conjunction with vitamin C.

If your gums bleed frequently when you brush your teeth, make sure you're getting enough rutin and hesperidin.

Anyone with a tendency to bruise easily will benefit from a C supplement with bioflavonoids, rutin, and hesperidin.

PABA [Para-aminobenzoic Acid]

FACTS:

Water soluble, one of the newer members of the B-complex family.

Usually measured in milligrams [mg.].

Can be synthesised in the body.

No RDA has yet been established.

Helps form folic acid and is important in the utilisation of protein.

Has important sun-screening properties.

Helps in the assimilation — and therefore the effectiveness — of pantothenic acid.

In experiments with animals, it has worked with pantothenic acid to restore grey hair to its natural colour.

WHAT IT CAN DO FOR YOU:

Used as an ointment it can protect against sunburn.

Reduce the pains of burns.

Keep skin healthy and smooth.

Help in delaying wrinkles.

Help to restore natural colour to your hair.

DEFICIENCY DISEASE:

Eczema.

BEST NATURAL SOURCES:

Liver, brewer's yeast, kidney, whole grains, rice, bran, wheat germ and molasses.

SUPPLEMENTS:

30 to 100 mg. are often included in good B-complex capsules as well as high-quality multi-vitamins.

Available in 30 to 1,000-mg strengths in regular and time-release form.

Doses most often used are 30 to 100 mg. three times a day.

TOXICITY:

No known toxic effects, but long-term programmes of high

dosages are not recommended.

Symptoms that might indicate an oversupply of PABA are usually nausea and vomiting.

ENEMIES:

Water, sulfa drugs, food-processing techniques, alcohol, oestrogen. [See Chapter XVIII.]

PERSONAL ADVICE:

Some people claim that the combination of folic acid and PABA has returned their greying hair to its natural colour. It has worked on animals, so it is certainly worth a try for anyone looking for an alternative to hair dye. For this purpose, 1,000 mg. [time release] daily for six days a week is a viable regimen.

If you tend to burn easily in the sun, use PABA as a protective ointment.

Many celebrities I know use PABA to prevent wrinkles. It doesn't eliminate them, but it certainly seems to keep them at bay for some people.

If you are taking penicillin, or any sulphur drug, your PABA intake should be increased through natural foods or supplements.

Vitamin T

There is very little known about this vitamin, except that it helps in blood coagulation and the forming of platelets. Because of these attributes it is important in warding off certain forms of anaemia and haemophilia. No RDA has been established, and there are no supplements for the public on the market. It is found in sesame seeds and egg yolks and there is no known toxicity.

Vitamin U

Even less is known about vitamin U than vitamin T. It is reputed to play an important role in healing ulcers, but medical opinions vary on this. It is found in raw cabbage and no known toxicity exists.

Some Questions About Chapter IV

I live in a big city and hear a lot about environmental pollution. I also hear a lot about how I need to take antioxidants. Could you tell me what antioxidants are and if I really need them?

Yes.

You really need them. Let me begin by saying that if you live in *any* major urban area today, you're breathing polluted air. Every year 200 million tons of potentially dangerous pollutants are released into the atmosphere.

With each breath you subject your lungs and body to a wide range of pollutants, and no part of you is immune. Antioxidants — vitamins A, C, E, and selenium, are nutrients that are capable of protecting other substances from oxidation. In other words, the free radicals (uncontrolled oxidations that damage cells) that are formed when we inhale pollutants are kept in check by antioxidants.

Vitamin A protects mucous membranes of mouth, nose, throat, and lungs. It also helps protect vitamin C from oxidation, which allows your C to work better.

Vitamin C fights bacterial infections and reduces the effects of allergy-producing substances. It also protects vitamins A, E, and some of the B complex from oxidation.

Vitamin E protects vitamins B and C from oxidation. It has the ability to unite with oxygen and prevent it from being converted into toxic peroxides. It acts as an antipollutant for the lungs.

Selenium and vitamin E must both be present to correct a deficiency in either. The levels of selenium in the blood of people in various cities has been found to bear a direct relationship to cancer mortality. The higher the levels of selenium, the lower the cancer death rate — and vice versa.

I've read that diets high in broccoli, brussels sprouts, and carrots can help reduce the risk of cancer, but I just hate these vegetables. What vitamins can I take instead?

You can get concentrated forms of cruciferous (cabbage,

broccoli, brussels sprouts, cauliflower) and carotene-rich (spinach and carrots) vegetables in tablet form. I'd advise taking these supplements daily. Since they are made from vegetables that are picked ripe, carefully washed, and quickly dehydrated without cooking — as well as being fortified with vitamins A, C, and E, beta-carotene and selenium — they'll provide you with optimal nutritional value.

Can you tell me how choline is helpful in the treatment of Alzheimer's disease?

Alzheimer's disease, which is a slow loss of mental faculties, and becoming so common among older individuals that many doctors are referring to it as "the disease of the '80s," seems to be caused by a depletion in central nervous system reserves of the neurotransmitter acetylcholine (not by a virus or aluminum, as previously suspected).

It has been found that patients with Alzheimer's syndrome are not only deficient in acetylcholine, but also the enzyme that catalyzes its production — choline acetyltransferase. Ingestion of more choline can apparently prevent existing acetylcholine from being broken down.

There is still no specific treatment for the disease, but it's been found that certain medications might worsen a patient's condition. For example, hypnotics such as *flurazepam* (DALMANE), drugs for heart disease, and those given for intestinal cramping.

V

Your Mineral Essentials

Calcium

FACTS:

There is more calcium in the body than any other mineral.

Calcium and phosphorus work together for healthy bones and teeth.

Calcium and magnesium work together for cardiovascular health.

Almost all of the body's calcium [two to three pounds] is found in the bones and teeth.

20 percent of an adult's bone calcium is reabsorbed and replaced every year. [New bone cells form as old ones break down.]

Calcium must exist in a two-to-one relationship with phosphorus.

In order for calcium to be absorbed, the body must have sufficient vitamin D.

For adults, 800 to 1,200 mg. is the RDA.

Calcium and iron are the two minerals most deficient in a woman's diet.

WHAT IT CAN DO FOR YOU:

Maintain strong bones and healthy teeth.

Keep your heart beating regularly.

Alleviate insomnia.

Help metabolise your body's iron.

Aid your nervous system, especially in impulse transmission.

DEFICIENCY DISEASE:

Rickets, osteomalacia, osteoporosis.

Best Natural Sources:

Milk and milk products, all cheeses, soyabeans, sardines, salmon, peanuts, walnuts, sunflower seeds, dried beans, green vegetables.

Supplements:

Most often available in 100- to 500-mg. tablets.

Bonemeal is a fairly common supplement, and a good source of the mineral though some people find calcium gluconate [a vegetarian source] or calcium lactate [a milk sugar derivative] easier to absorb. [Gluconate is more potent than lactate.]

The best form is chelated calcium tablets.

Many good multivitamin and mineral preparations include calcium.

When combined with magnesium, the ratio should be twice as much calcium as magnesium. Dolomite is a natural form of calcium and magnesium, and no vitamin D is needed for assimilation. Five dolomite tablets are equivalent to 750 mg. of calcium.

Doses most often used are 800 to 2,000 mg. per day.

Toxicity:

Excessive daily intake of over 2,000 mg. might lead to hypercalcemia. [See Chapter XXIII "Cautions."]

Enemies:

Large quantities of fat, oxalic acid [found in chocolate and rhubarb], and phytic acid [found in grains] are capable of preventing proper calcium absorption.

Personal Advice:

If you are afflicted with backaches, dolomite, chelated calcium, or bonemeal supplements might help.

Menstrual-cramp sufferers can often find relief by increasing their calcium intake.

Teenagers who suffer from "growing pains" will usually find that they disappear with an increase in calcium consumption.

Hypoglycaemics could use more calcium.

Chlorine

FACTS:

Regulates the blood's alkaline-acid balance.
Works with sodium and potassium in a compound form.
Aids in the cleaning of body wastes by helping the liver to function.
No dietary allowance has been established, but if your daily salt intake is average, you are getting enough.

WHAT IT CAN DO FOR YOU:

Aid in digestion.
Help keep you limber.

DEFICIENCY DISEASE:

Loss of hair and teeth.

BEST NATURAL SOURCES:

Table salt, kelp, olives.

SUPPLEMENTS:

Most good multimineral preparations include it.

TOXICITY:

Over 15 g. can cause unpleasant side effects.

PERSONAL ADVICE:

If you have chlorine in your drinking water, you aren't getting all the vitamin E you think. [Chlorinated water destroys vitamin E.]
Anyone who drinks chlorinated water would be well advised to eat yoghurt — a good way to replace the intestinal bacteria the chlorine destroys.

Chromium

FACTS:

Works with insulin in the metabolism of sugar.

Helps bring protein to where it's needed.

No official dietary allowance has been established, but 90 mcg. is an average adult intake.

As you get older, you retain less chromium in your body.

WHAT IT CAN DO FOR YOU:

Aid growth.
Help prevent and lower high blood pressure.
Works as a deterrent for diabetes.

DEFICIENCY DISEASE:

A suspected factor in arteriosclerosis and diabetes.

BEST NATURAL SOURCES:

Meat, shellfish, chicken, corn oil, clams, brewer's yeast.

SUPPLEMENTS:

May be found in the better multimineral preparations.

TOXICITY:

No known toxicity.

PERSONAL ADVICE:

If you are low in chromium (a hair analysis would show this) you might try a zinc supplement. For some reason, chelated zinc seems to substitute well for deficient chromium.

Cobalt

FACTS:

A mineral that is part of vitamin B_{12}.
Usually measured in micrograms [mcg.].
Essential for red blood cells.
Must be obtained from food sources.
No daily allowance has been set for this mineral, and only very small amounts are necessary in the diet [usually no more than 8 mcg.].

WHAT IT CAN DO FOR YOU:

Stave off anaemia.

DEFICIENCY DISEASE:

Anaemia.

BEST NATURAL SOURCES:

Meat, kidney, liver, milk, oysters, clams.

SUPPLEMENTS:

Rarely found in supplement form.

TOXICITY:

No known toxicity.

ENEMIES:

Whatever is antagonistic to B_{12}.

PERSONAL ADVICE:

If you're a strict vegetarian, you are much more likely to be deficient in this mineral than someone who includes meat and shellfish in his or her diet.

Copper

FACTS:

Required to convert the body's iron into haemoglobin.
Can reach the bloodstream fifteen minutes after ingestion.
Makes the amino acid tyrosine usable, allowing it to work as the pigmenting factor for hair and skin.
Present in cigarettes, birth-control pills, and automobile pollution.
Essential for the utilisation of vitamin C.
The RDA has not been set by the National Research Council, but 2 mg. for adults is suggested.

WHAT IT CAN DO FOR YOU:

Keep your energy up by aiding in effective iron absorption.

DEFICIENCY DISEASE:

Anaemia, edema.

BEST NATURAL SOURCES:

Dried beans, peas, whole wheat, prunes, calf and beef liver, shrimp, and most seafood.

SUPPLEMENTS:

Usually available in multivitamin and mineral supplements in 2-mg. doses.

TOXICITY:

Rare. [See Chapter XXIII "Cautions."]

ENEMIES:

Not easily destroyed.

PERSONAL ADVICE:

As essential as copper is, I rarely suggest special supplementation. An excess seems to lower zinc level and produce insomnia, hair loss, irregular menses, and depression.

If you eat enough whole-grain products, and fresh green leafy vegetables, as well as liver, you don't have to worry about your copper intake.

Fluorine

FACTS:

Part of the synthetic compound sodium fluoride [the type added to drinking water] and calcium fluoride [a natural substance].

Decreases chances of dental caries, though too much can discolour teeth.

No RDA has been established, but most people get about 1 mg. daily from fluoridated drinking water.

WHAT IT CAN DO FOR YOU:

Reduce tooth decay.

Strengthen bones.

DEFICIENCY DISEASE:

Tooth decay.

BEST NATURAL SOURCES:

Fluoridated drinking water, seafoods, and gelatin.

SUPPLEMENTS:

Not ordinarily found in multimineral supplements.

TOXICITY:

20 to 80 mg. per day.

ENEMIES:

Aluminium salts of fluorine.

PERSONAL ADVICE:

Don't take additional fluoride unless it is prescribed by a physician or dentist.

Iodine [Iodide]

FACTS:

Two-thirds of the body's iodine is in the thyroid gland.

Since the thyroid gland controls metabolism, and iodine influences the thyroid, an under-supply of this mineral can result in slow mental reaction, weight gain, and lack of energy.

The RDA, as established by the National Research Council, is 80 to 150 mcg. for adults [1 mcg. per kilogram of body weight] and 125 to 150 mcg. for pregnant and lactating women respectively.

WHAT IT CAN DO FOR YOU:

Help you with dieting by burning excess fat.
Promote proper growth.
Give you more energy.
Improve mental alacrity.

77

Promote healthy hair, nails, skin, and teeth.

DEFICIENCY DISEASE:

Goitre, hypothyroidism.

BEST NATURAL SOURCES:

Kelp, vegetables grown in iodine-rich soil, onions, and all seafood.

SUPPLEMENTS:

Available in multimineral and high-potency vitamin supplements in doses of 0.15 mg.
Natural kelp is a good source of supplemental iodine.

TOXICITY:

No known toxicity from natural iodine, though iodine as a drug can be harmful if prescribed incorrectly. [See Chapter XXIII "Cautions."]

ENEMIES:

Food processing, nutrient-poor soil.

PERSONAL ADVICE:

Aside from kelp, and the iodine included in multimineral and vitamin preparations, I don't recommended additional supplements unless you're advised by a doctor to take them.
If you use salt and live where iodine-poor soil is common, make sure the salt is iodised.
If you are inclined to eat excessive amounts of raw cabbage, you might *not* be getting the iodine you need, because there are elements in the cabbage that prevent proper utilisation of the iodine. This being the case, you should consider a kelp supplement.

Iron.

FACTS:

Essential and required for life, necessary for the production of haemoglobin [red blood corpuscles], myoglobin [red pigment in muscles], and certain enzymes.

Iron and calcium are the two major dietary deficiencies of women.

Only about 8 per cent of your total iron intake is absorbed and actually enters your bloodstream.

An average 150-pound adult has about 4 g. of iron in his or her body. Haemoglobin, which accounts for most of the iron, is recycled and reutilised as blood cells are replaced every 120 days. Iron bound to protein [ferritin] is stored in the body, as is tissue iron [present in myoglobin] in very small amounts.

The RDA, according to the National Research Council, is 10 to 18 mg. for adults, and 18 mg. for pregnant and lactating women.

In one month, women lose almost twice as much iron as men.

Copper, cobalt, manganese, and vitamin C are necessary to assimilate iron. Iron is necessary for proper metabolisation of B vitamins.

WHAT IT CAN DO FOR YOU:

Aid growth.
Promote resistance to disease.
Prevent fatigue.
Cure and prevent iron-deficiency anaemia.
Bring back good skin tone.

DEFICIENCY DISEASE:

Iron-deficiency anaemia.

BEST NATURAL SOURCES:

Pork liver, beef kidney, heart and liver, farina, raw clams, dried peaches, red meat, egg yolks, oysters, nuts, beans, asparagus, molasses, oatmeal.

SUPPLEMENTS:

The most assimilable form of iron is hydrolysed-protein chelate, which means organic iron that has been processed for fastest assimilation. This form is nonconstipating and easy on sensitive systems.

Ferrous sulphate, inorganic iron, appears in many vitamin and mineral supplements and can destroy vitamin E [they should be taken at least eight hours apart]. Check labels; many formulas contain ferrous sulphate.

Supplements with organic iron — ferrous gluconate, ferrous fumerate, ferrous citrate, or ferrous peptonate — do not neutralise vitamin E. They are available in a wide variety of doses, usually up to 320 mg.

TOXICITY:

Rare in healthy, normal individuals. Excessive doses, thought, can be a hazard for children. [See Chapter XXIII "Cautions."]

ENEMIES:

Phosphoproteins in eggs and phytates in unleavened whole wheat reduce iron availability to body.

PERSONAL ADVICE:

If you are a woman, I recommend an iron supplement. Check the label on your multivitamin or mineral preparation and see what you are already getting and guide yourself accordingly. [Remember, if the iron in your preparation is ferrous sulphate, you're losing your vitamin E.]

Keep your iron supplements out of the reach of children.

Coffee drinkers, as well as tea drinkers, be aware that if you consume large quantities of either beverage you are most likely inhibiting your iron absorption.

Magnesium

FACTS:

Necessary for calcium and vitamin-C metabolism, as well as that of phosphorus, sodium, and potassium.

Measured in milligrams [mg.].

Essential for effective nerve and muscle functioning.

Important for converting blood sugar into energy.

Known as the antistress mineral.

Alcoholics are usually deficient.

Adults need 300 to 400 mg. daily, slightly more for pregnant

80

and lactating women, according to the US National Research Council.

The human body contains approximately 21 g. of magnesium.

WHAT IT CAN DO FOR YOU:

Aid in fighting depression.
Promote a healthier cardiovascular system and help prevent heart attacks.
Keep teeth healthier.
Help prevent calcium deposits, kidney and gallstones.
Bring relief from indigestion.

DEFICIENCY DISEASE:

[See Chapter VIII]

BEST NATURAL SOURCES:

Figs, lemons, grapefruit, yellow corn, almonds, nuts, seeds, dar-green vegetables, apples.

SUPPLEMENTS:

Dolomite, which has magnesium and calcium in perfect balance [half as much magnesium as calcium], is a fine magnesium supplement.
Available in multivitamin and mineral preparations [best if they are chelated].
Can be purchased as magnesium oxide. 250-mg. strength equals 150 mg. per tablet.
Commonly available in 133.3-mg. strengths and taken four times a day.
Supplements of magnesium should not be taken after meals, since the mineral does neutralise stomach acidity.

TOXICITY:

Large amounts, over an extended period of time, can be toxic if your calcium and phosphorus intakes are high. [See Chapter XXIII "Cautions."]

ENEMIES:

Diuretics, alcohol. [See Chapter XXIII.]

If you are a drinker, I suggest you increase your intake of magnesium.

Women who are on the pill or taking oestrogen in any form would be well advised to take larger amounts of magnesium.

If you are a heavy consumer of nuts, seeds, and green vegetables, you probably get ample magnesium — as does anyone who lives in an area with hard water.

Magnesium works best with vitamin A, calcium and phosphorus.

Manganese

FACTS:

Helps activate enzymes, necessary for the body's proper use of biotin, B_1, and vitamin C.

Needed for normal bone structure.

Measured in milligrams [mg.].

Important in the formation of thyroxin, the principal hormone of the thyroid gland.

Necessary for the proper digestion and utilisation of food.

No official daily allowance has been set, but 2.5 to 7 mg. is generally accepted to be the average adult requirement.

Important for reproduction and normal central nervous system function.

WHAT IT CAN DO FOR YOU:

Help eliminate fatigue.
Aid in muscle reflexes.
Improve memory.
Reduce nervous irritability.

DEFICIENCY DISEASE:

Ataxia.

BEST NATURAL SOURCES:

Nuts, green leafy vegetables, peas, beets, egg yolks, whole-grain cereals.

SUPPLEMENTS:

Most often found in multivitamin and mineral combinations in dosages of 1 to 9 mg.

TOXICITY:

Rare, except from industrial sources. [See Chapter XXIII "Cautions."]

ENEMIES:

Large intakes of calcium and phosphorus will inhibit absorption.

PERSONAL ADVICE:

If you suffer from recurrent dizziness, you might try adding more manganese to your diet.

I advise absent-minded people, or anyone with memory problems, to make sure they are getting enough of this mineral.

Heavy milk drinkers and meat eaters need increased manganese.

Molybdenum

FACTS:

Aids in carbohydrate and fat metabolism.

A vital part of the enzyme responsible for iron utilisation.

No dietary allowance has been set, but the estimated daily intake of 45 to 500 mcg. has generally been accepted as the adequate human requirement.

WHAT IT CAN DO FOR YOU:

Help in preventing anaemia.
Promote general well-being.

DEFICIENCY DISEASE:

None known.

BEST NATURAL SOURCES:

Dark-green leafy vegetables, whole grains, legumes.

No ordinarily available.

Toxicity:

Rare, but 5 to 10 parts per million has been considered toxic.

Personal Advice:

As important as molybdenum is, there seems no need for supplementation unless all the food you consume comes from nutrient-deficient soil.

Phosphorus

Facts:

Present in every cell in the body.
Vitamin D and calcium are essential to proper phosphorus functioning.
Calcium and phosphorus should be balanced two to one to work correctly [twice as much calcium as phosphorus].
Involved in virtually all physiological chemical reactions.
Necessary for normal bone and tooth structure.
Niacin cannot be assimilated without phosphorus.
Important for heart regularity.
Essential for normal kidney functioning.
Needed for the transference of nerve impulses.
The RDA is 800 to 1,200 mg. for adults, the higher levels for pregnant and lactating women.

What It Can Do For You:

Aid in growth and body repair.
Provide energy and vigour by helping in the metabolisation of fats and starches.
Lessen the pain of arthritis.
Promote healthy gums and teeth.

Deficiency Disease:

Rickets, pyorrhoea.

BEST NATURAL SOURCES:

Fish, poultry, meat, whole grains, eggs, nuts, seeds.

SUPPLEMENTS:

Bonemeal is a fine natural source of phosphorus. [Make sure vitamin D has been added to help assimilation.]

TOXICITY:

No known toxicity. [See Chapter XXIII "Cautions."]

ENEMIES:

Too much iron, aluminium, and magnesium can render phosphorus ineffective.

PERSONAL ADVICE:

When you get too much phosphorus, you throw off your mineral balance and decrease your calcium. Our diets are usually high in phosphorus — since it does occur in almost every natural food — and therefore calcium deficiencies are frequent. Be aware of this and adjust your diet accordingly.

If you're over forty, you should cut down on your weekly meat consumption and eat more leafy vegetables and drink milk. The reason for this is that after forty our kidneys don't help excrete excess phosphorus, and calcium is again depleted. Be on the lookout for foods preserved with phosphates and consider that as part of your phosphorus intake.

Potassium

FACTS:

Works with sodium to regulate the body's water balance and normalise heart rhythms. [Potassium works inside the cells, sodium works just outside them.]

Nerve and muscle functions suffer when the sodium-potassium balance is off.

Hypoglycaemia [low blood sugar] causes potassium loss, as does a long, fast or severe diarrhoea.

No dietary allowance has been set, but approximately 900 mg.

is considered a healthy daily intake.

Both mental and physical stress can lead to a potassium deficiency.

WHAT IT CAN DO FOR YOU:

Aid in clear thinking by sending oxygen to brain.
Help dispose of body wastes.
Assist in reducing blood pressure.
Aid in allergy treatment.

DEFICIENCY DISEASE:

Edema, hypoglycaemia.

BEST NATURAL SOURCES:

Citrus fruits, watercress, all green leafy vegetables, mint leaves, sunflower seeds, bananas, potatoes.

SUPPLEMENTS:

Available in most high-potency multivitamin and multimineral preparations.

Inorganic potassium "salts" are the sulphate [alum], the chloride, the oxide and carbonate. Organic potassium refers to the gluconate, the citrate, the fumerate.

Can be bought separately as potassium gluconate in dosages up to nearly 600 mg.

TOXICITY:

25 g. of potassium chloride can cause toxicity. [See Chapter XXIII "Cautions."]

ENEMIES:

Alcohol, coffee, sugar, diuretics.

PERSONAL ADVICE:

If you drink large amounts of coffee, you might find that the fatigue you're fighting is due to the potassium loss you're suffering from.

Heavy drinkers and anyone with a hungry sweet tooth should be aware that their potassium levels are probably low.

If you have low blood sugar, you are likely to be losing potassium while retaining water. And if you take a diuretic, you'll lose even more potassium. Watch your diet, increase your green vegetables, and take enough magnesium to regain your mineral balance.

Losing weight on a low-carbohydrate diet might not be the only thing you're losing. Chances are your potassium level is down. Watch our for weakness and poor reflexes.

Selenium

FACTS:

Vitamin E and selenium are synergistic. This means that the two together are stronger than the sum of the equal parts.

Both vitamin E and selenium are antioxidants, preventing or at least slowing down aging and hardening of tissues through oxidation.

Males appear to have a greater need for selenium. Almost half their body's supply concentrates in the testicles and portions of the seminal ducts adjacent to the prostate gland. Also, selenium is lost in the semen.

No official dietary allowance has yet been set for this mineral, but the general dosage is between 50 and 100 mcg. It is not advisable to exceed 200 mcg. daily.

WHAT IT CAN DO FOR YOU:

Aid in keeping youthful elasticity in tissues.
Alleviate hot flushes and menopausal distress.
Help in treatment and prevention of dandruff.
Possibly neutralise certain carcinogens and provide protection from some cancers.

DEFICIENCY DISEASE:

Premature stamina loss.

BEST NATURAL SOURCES:

Wheat germ, bran, tuna fish, onions, tomatoes, broccoli.

Available in small microgram doses. 25 to 50 mcg. is most often used.

Also available combined with vitamin E and other antioxidants.

Natural foods supply sufficient amounts when eaten regularly.

TOXICITY:

Doses above 5 parts per million can be toxic.

ENEMIES:

Food-processing techniques.

PERSONAL ADVICE:

Selenium was discovered only a little more than twenty years ago. We've just begun to recognise its importance in human nutrition. Until more is known, I advise taking only moderate supplements.

Sodium

FACTS:

Sodium and potassium were discovered together and both found to be essential for normal growth.

High intakes of sodium [salt] will result in a depletion of potassium.

Diets high in sodium usually account for many instances of high blood pressure.

There is no official allowance, but a daily single gram of sodium chloride has been suggested for each kilogram of water drunk. Sodium aids in keeping calcium and other minerals in the blood soluble.

WHAT IT CAN DO FOR YOU:

Aid in preventing heat prostration or sunstroke.
Help your nerves and muscles function properly.

DEFICIENCY DISEASE:

Impaired carbohydrates digestion, possibly neuralgia.

BEST NATURAL SOURCES:

Salt, shellfish, carrots, beets, artichokes, dried beef, brains, kidney, bacon.

SUPPLEMENTS:

Rarely needed, but if so, kelp is a safe and nutritive supplement.

TOXICITY:

Over 14 g. of sodium chloride daily can produce toxic effects.

PERSONAL ADVICE:

If you think you don't each much salt, you are probably mistaken.

If you have high blood pressure, cut down on your sodium intake by reading the labels on the foods you buy. Look for SALT, SODIUM, or the chemical symbol *Na*.

Adding sodium to your diet is as easy as a shake of salt, but subtracting it can be difficult. Avoid luncheon meats, frankfurters, salted cured meats such as ham, bacon, corned beef, as well as condiments — ketchup, chili sauce, soya sauce, mustard. Don't use baking powder or baking soda in cooking.

Sulphur

FACTS:

Essential for healthy hair, skin and nails.

Helps maintain oxygen balance necessary for proper brain function.

Works with B-complex vitamins for basic body metabolism, and is part of tissue-building amino acids.

Aids the liver in bile secretion.

No RDA has been set, but a diet sufficient in protein will generally be sufficient in sulphur.

WHAT IT CAN DO FOR YOU:

Tone up skin and make hair more lustrous.
Help fight bacterial infections.

DEFICIENCY DISEASE:

None known.

BEST NATURAL SOURCES:

Lean beef, dried beans, fish, eggs, cabbage.

SUPPLEMENTS:

Not readily available as a food supplement.
Can be found in topical ointments and creams for skin problems.

TOXICITY:

No known toxicity from organic sulphur, but ill effects may occur from large amounts of inorganic sulphur.

PERSONAL ADVICE:

If you're getting enough protein in your daily meals, you are, most likely, getting enough sulphur.
Sulphur creams and ointments have been remarkably successful in treating a variety of skin problems. Check the ingredients in the preparation you are now using. There are many fine natural preparations available at healthfood centres.

Vanadium

FACTS:

Inhibits the formation of cholesterol in blood vessels.
No dietary allowance set.

WHAT IT CAN DO FOR YOU:

Aid in preventing heart attacks.

DEFICIENCY DISEASE:

None known.

Fish.

Not available.

Toxicity:

Can easily be toxic if taken in synthetic form.

Personal Advice:

This is not one of the minerals that needs to be supplemented. A good fish dinner will supply you with the vanadium you need.

Zinc

Facts:

Zinc acts as a traffic policeman, directing and overseeing the efficient flow of body processes, the maintenance of enzyme system and cells.

Essential for protein synthesis.

Governs the contractibility of muscles.

Helps in the formation of insulin.

Important for blood stability and in maintaining the body's acid-alkaline balance.

Exerts a normalising effect on the prostate and is important in the development of all reproductive organs.

New studies indicate its importance in brain function and the treatment of schizophrenia.

Strong evidence of its requirement for the synthesis of DNA.

The RDA, as set by the U.S. National Research Council, is 15 mg. for adults [slightly higher allowances for pregnant and lactating women].

Excessive sweating can cause a loss of as much as 3 mg. of zinc per day.

Most zinc in foods is lost in processing, or never exists in substantial amount due to nutrient-poor soil.

91

What It Can Do For You:

Accelerate healing time for internal and external wounds.
Get rid of white spots on the fingernails.
Help eliminate loss of taste.
Aid in the treatment of infertility.
Help avoid prostate problems.
Promote growth and mental alertness.
Help decrease cholesterol deposits.

Deficiency Disease:

Possibly prostatic hypertrophy [non-cancerous enlargement of the prostate gland], arteriosclerosis.

Best Natural Sources:

Round steak, lamb chops, pork loin, wheat germ, brewer's yeast, pumpkin seeds, eggs, nonfat dry milk, ground mustard.

Supplements:

Available in all good multivitamin and multimineral preparations.

Can be bought as zinc-sulphate or zinc-gluconate tablets in doses ranging from 15 to over 300 mg. Both zinc sulphate and zinc gluconate seem to be equally effective, but zinc gluconate appears to be more easily tolerated.

Chelated zinc is the best way to take zinc.

Zinc is also available in combination with vitamin C, magnesium, and the B-complex vitamins.

Toxicity:

Virtually nontoxic, except when there is an excessive intake and the food ingested has been stored in galvanised containers. Doses over 150 mg. are not recommended. [See Chapter XXIII "Cautions."]

Personal Advice:

You need higher intakes of zinc if you are taking large amounts of vitamin B_6. This is also true if you are an alcoholic or a diabetic.

Men with prostate problems — and without them — would be well advised to keep their zinc levels up.

I have seen success in cases of impotence with a supplement programme of B_6 and zinc.

Elderly people, concerned about senility, might find a zinc and manganese supplement beneficial.

If you are bothered by irregular menses, you might try a zinc supplement before resorting to hormone treatment to establish regularity.

Remember, if you are adding zinc to your diet, you will increase the need for vitamin A. Zinc works best with vitamin A, calcium and phosphorus.

Water

FACTS:

The simple truth is that this is our most important nutrient. One-half to three-quarters of the body's weight is water.

A human being can live for weeks without food, but only a few days without water.

Water is the basic solvent for all the products of digestion.

Essential for removing wastes.

There is no specific dietary allowance since water loss varies with climate, situations, and individuals, but under ordinary circumstances six glasses daily is considered healthy.

Regulates body temperature.

WHAT IT CAN DO FOR YOU:

Keep all your bodily functions functioning.
Aid in dieting by depressing appetite before meals.
Help prevent constipation.

DEFICIENCY DISEASE:

Dehydration.

BEST NATURAL SOURCES:

Drinking water, juices, fruits, and vegetables.

All drinkable liquids can substitute for only daily water requirements.

Toxicity:

No known toxicity, but an intake of one and a half gallons [that's sixteen to twenty-four glasses] in about an hour could be dangerous for an adult. It could kill an infant.

Personal Advice:

I advise six to eight glasses of water daily, to be drunk a half hour before meals, for anyone who's dieting.

If you're running a fever, be sure to drinks lots of water to prevent dehydration and to flush systems of wastes.

If you live in an area where there is hard water, you're probably getting more calcium and magnesium than you think.

VI

Protein — and the Amazing Amino Acids

The Protein Amino Acid Connection

Protein is a life necessity in the diet of man and all animals. Actually, though, it is not protein itself that is required, but the amino acids which are the building blocks of protein. If any essential amino acid is low or missing, the effectiveness of all the others will be proportionately reduced.

Amino acids, which bonded with nitrogen form thousands of different proteins, are not only the units from which proteins are formed, but are also the end products of protein digestion.

There are twenty-two known amino acids. Eight of these are called *essential amino acids*. These essential amino acids *cannot*, like the others, be manufactured by the human body and *must* be obtained from food or supplements. A ninth amino acid, histidine, is considered essential *only* for infants and children.

THE 22 AMINO ACIDS
(Essential amino acids are marked with asterisks.)

Alanine	*Leucine
Arginine	*Lysine
Asparagine	*Methionine
Aspartic acid	Ornithine
Cysteine	*Phenylalanine
Cystine	Proline
Glutamic acid	Serine
Glutamine	*Threonine
Glycine	*Tryptophan
*Histidine	Tyrosine
*Isoleucine	*Valine

In order for the body to use effectively and synthesize protein, all the essential amino acids must be present and in the proper proportions. Even the temporary absence of a single essential amino acid can adversely affect protein synthesis. In fact, whatever essential amino acid is low or missing will proportionately reduce the effectiveness of all the others.

How Much Protein Do You Need, Really?

Everyone's protein requirements differ, depending on a variety of factors including health, age, and size. Actually, the larger and younger you are, the more you need. To estimate your own personal daily recommended allowance, see the chart below.

AGE	1–3	4–6	7–10	11–14	15–18	19+
POUND KEY	0.82	0.68	0.55	0.45	0.40	0.36

Find the pound key under your age group.
Multiply that number by your weight.
The result will be your daily protein requirement in grams.

Example: You weigh 100 pounds and are thirty-three years old.

Your pound key is 0.36.

0.36 × 100 = 36g. — your daily protein requirement.

An average minimum protein requirement is around 45 g. a day. That's 15 g. or about half an ounce per meal. Make sure you get enough at breakfast.

Types of Protein — What's the Difference?

All proteins are not the same, though they're manufactured from the same twenty-two amino acids. They have different functions and work in different areas of the body.

There are basically two types of protein — complete protein and incomplete protein.

Complete protein provides the proper balance of the eight necessary amino acids that build tissues, and is found in foods of animal origin such as meats, poultry, seafood, eggs, milk, and cheese.

Incomplete protein lacks certain essential amino acids and is not used efficiently when eaten alone. However, when it is combined with small amounts of animal-source protein, it becomes complete. It is found in seeds, nuts, peas, grains, and beans.

Mixing complete and incomplete proteins can give you better nutrition than either one alone. A good rice-and beans dish with some cheese can be just as nourishing, less expensive, and lower in fat than a steak.

Protein Myths

A lot of people seem to think that protein is non-fattening. This misconception has frustrated many a determined dieter who forgoes bread but eats healthy portions of steak and wonders where the weight is coming from. The fact is

1 g. protein	= 4 calories
1 g. carbohydrate	= 4 calories
1 g. fat	= 9 calories

In other words, protein and carbohydrate have the same gram-for-gram calorie count.

It is also thought that protein can burn up fat. This is another erroneous assumption that leaves dieters staring incomprehensibly at their scales. It just is not true that the more protein you eat the thinner you'll get. And, believe it or not, one homemade beef taco or a slice of cheese pizza will give you more protein than two eggs or four slices of bacon or even a whole cup of milk. (Of course, if pizza is made with all sorts of additives, you're better off taking a cut in protein and sticking with the eggs.)

Protein Supplements

Two tablespoons of supplement equal the protein in a three-ounce steak. For anyone who isn't able to get their daily protein requirement from whole food, protein supplements are helpful. The best formulas are derived from soybeans, which contain all the essential amino acids. They come in liquid and powdered form, are available without carbohydrates or fats, and generally supply about 26 g. of protein an ounce (two tablespoons). That would be about the same amount of protein you get from a three-ounce T-bone.

Supplements can easily be added to beverages and foods. Texturized vegetable protein can be added to ground beef to extend and enhance hamburgers, which will be more economical and better for you because of the cut in saturated fat.

Amino Acid Supplements

Free-form amino acids are now available in balanced formulas or as individual supplements, because so many have been found to offer specific health-enhancing properties — from improving the immune system to reducing dependence on drugs.

It's wise, when taking amino acid supplements, to take also the major vitamins that are involved in their metabolism, for instance: Vitamins B_6, B_{12}, and niacin. And if you're going to take an amino acid formula, make sure it's well-balanced. *Read the label!* For protein synthesis to occur, there must be the balance between "essential" and "nonessential" amino acids, and the essentials in proper proportion to one another. (Lysine should be in a 2:1 ratio to methionine, 3:1 to tryptophan, and so on. When in doubt, ask your pharmacist or consult a reliable nutritionist. What you want is a formula that's modelled after naturally occurring proteins so that you can get the proper therapeutic value.

CAUTION: It's dangerous for any supplement to be used in place of food on a regular basis or taken in megadoses without the advice of a physician. Always keep them out of the reach of children.

Tryptophan

Tryptophan is an essential amino acid that's used by the brain — along with vitamin B_6, niacin (or niacinamide), and magnesium — to produce serotonin, a neurotransmitter that carries messages between the brain and one of the body's biochemical mechanisms of sleep.

WHAT IT CAN DO FOR YOU:

Help induce natural sleep.
Reduce pain sensitivity.
Act as a non-drug antidepressant.
Aid in reducing anxiety and tension.
Help relieve some symptoms of alcohol-related body chemistry disorders and aid in control of alcoholism.

BEST NATURAL SOURCES:

Cottage cheese, milk, meat, fish, turkey, bananas, dried dates, peanuts, all protein-rich foods.

SUPPLEMENT GUIDE:

L-tryptophan comes in tablets of 250 mg. to 667 mg. strengths. When used as a relaxant, it should be taken during the day between meals, with juice or water — no milk or other protein.

As a sleep inducer, L-tryptophan works best when taken in a 500 mg. dose, along with vitamin B_6 100 mg., niacinamide 100 mg., and chelated magnesium 130 mg., 1½ hours before bedtime. (Again, these should be taken with juice or water — no protein.)

Many doctors, including Dr. David Bressler, formerly of The Pain Control Centre at the University of California, suggest taking an additional tryptophan tablet ½ hour before bedtime to help sleeping all through the night.

CAUTION: Single dosages exceeding 2 grams are not recommended, even though successful tests at the Maryland Psychiatric Research Centre have shown that there is no danger of tryptophan addiction or overdose. (Because tryptophan is a natural part of our physical makeup, the body doesn't have to change any function to make use of it as it does with drugs.)

PERSONAL ADVICE AND COMMENTS:

If you are taking L-tryptophan, be sure that you're also taking a complete balanced B-complex formula (50–100 mg. of B_1, B_2 and B_6) with your morning and evening meals.

You can prolong the relaxant effects of tryptophan by taking it in a 2-to-1 ratio with niacinamide (twice as much tryptophan as niacinamide). Niacinamide has an antidepressant effect of its own.

Phenylalanine

Phenylalanine is an essential amino acid that is a neurotransmitter, a chemical that transmits its signals between the nerve cells and the brain. In the body it's turned into noradrenaline and dopamine, excitatory transmitters, which promote alertness and vitality. Do not confuse it with DL-phenylalanine.

WHAT IT CAN DO FOR YOU:

> Reduce hunger.
> Increase sexual interest.
> Improve memory and mental alertness.
> Alleviate depression.

BEST NATURAL SOURCES:

All protein-rich foods, bread stuffing, soy products, cottage cheese, dry skim milk, almonds, peanuts, lima beans, pumpkin and sesame seeds.

Available in 250–500 mg. tablets. For appetite control, tablets should be taken one hour before meals with juice or water (no protein).

For general alertness and vitality, tablets should be taken between meals, but again with water or juice (no protein).

CAUTION: Phenylalanine is contraindicated during pregnancy and for people with phenylketonuria or skin cancer.

Personal Advice And Comments:

Before resorting to prescription or 'recreational' drugs, I'd advise giving this natural "upper" a chance. Keep in mind, though, that it cannot be metabolized if you are deficient in vitamin C.

Phenylalanine is nonaddictive, *but it can raise blood pressure!* If you are hypertensive or have a heart condition, I'd advise checking with your doctor before using phenylalanine. In most cases, persons, with high blood pressure are able to take phenylalanine *after* meals, but consult your doctor first.

DL-Phenylalanine (DLPA)

This form of the essential amino acid phenylalanine is a mixture of equal parts of D (synthetic) and L (natural) phenylalanine. By producing and activating morphinelike hormones called *endorphins*, it intensifies and prolongs the body's own natural pain-killing response to injury, accident, and disease.

Certain enzyme systems in the body continually destroy endorphins, but DL-phenylalanine effectively inhibits these enzymes, allowing the pain-killing endorphins to do their job. Many people who do not respond to conventional pain-killers *do* respond to DLPA.

People who suffer from chronic pain have lower levels of endorphin activity in their blood and cerebro-spinal fluid. Since DLPA can restore normal endorphin levels, it can thereby assist the body in reducing pain naturally — without the use of drugs.

Moreover, because DLPA is capable of selective pain-blocking, it can effectively alleviate chronic long-term discomfort while leaving the body's natural defense mechanisms for short-term acute pain (burns, cuts, etc.) unhindered.

The effect of DLPA often equals or exceeds that of morphine and other opiate derivatives, but DLPA differs from prescription and over-the-counter medicines in that —

it is nonaddictive;

pain relief becomes *more* effective over time (without development of tolerance);

it has strong anti-depressant action;

it can provide continuous pain relief for up to a month without additional medication;

it's non-toxic;

it can be combined with any other medication or therapy to increase benefits without adverse interactions.

What It Can Do For You:

Act as a natural pain-killer for conditions such as whiplash, osteoarthritis, rheumatoid arthritis, lower back pain, migraines, leg and muscle cramps, postoperative pain, and neuralgia.

Supplement Guide:

DL-phenylalanine is generally available in 375 mg. tablets. Correct dosages vary according to the individual's own experience of pain.

Six tablets per day (two tablets taken approximately 15 minutes before each meal) is the best way to begin a DLPA regimen. Pain relief should occur within the first four days, though it may, in some cases, take as long as three to four weeks. If no substantial relief is noticed in the first three weeks, double the initial dosage for an additional two to three weeks. If treatment is still not effective, discontinue the regimen. It's been found that 5–15% of users do not respond to DLPA's analgesic properties.)

CAUTION: DLPA is contraindicated during pregnancy and for people with phenylketonuria. Because it elevates blood pressure, people with heart conditions or hypertension should check with a doctor before starting any DLPA regimen. Usually, though, it's allowed if taken *after* meals.

On a DLPA regimen, pain usually diminishes within the first week. Dosages can then be reduced gradually until a minimum requirement is determined. Whatever yours turns out to be, doses should be regularly spaced throughout the day.

Some people require only one week of DLPA supplements a month; others need it on a continuous basis. I found it interesting to discover that many people who do not respond to conventional prescription pain-killers *do* respond to DLPA.)

Lysine

This essential amino acid is vital in the makeup of critical body proteins. It's needed for growth, tissue repair, and the production of antibodies, hormones, and enzymes.

What It Can Do For You:

Help reduce the incidence of and/or prevent herpes infection.
Promote better concentration.
Properly utilize fatty acids needed for energy production.
Aid in alleviating some fertility problems.

Best Natural Sources:

Fish, milk, lima beans, meat, cheese, yeast, eggs, soy products, all protein-rich foods.

Supplement Guide:

L-lysine is generally available in 500 mg. capsules. The usual dosage is 1–2 capsules daily at mealtime.

Personal Advice And Comments:

If you're often tired, unable to concentrate, prone to blood-shot eyes, nausea, dizziness, hair loss, and anaemia, you could have a lysine deficiency.

Older persons, particularly men, require more lysine than younger ones.

Lysine is lacking in certain cereal proteins such as gliadin (from wheat) and zein (from corn). Supplementation of wheat-based foods with lysine improves their protein quality.

If you have herpes, lysine supplements in doses of 3–6 grams daily — plus lysine-rich foods — are strongly recommended.

Arginine

This amino acid is necessary for the normal function of the pituitary gland. Along with ornithine, phenylalanine, and other neuro chemicals, arginine is required for the synthesis and release of the pituitary gland's growth hormone. The need for arginine is especially great in males, since seminal fluids contain as much as 80% of this protein building-block, and a deficiency could lead to infertility.

WHAT IT CAN DO FOR YOU:

Increase sperm count in males.
Aid in immune response and healing of wounds.
Help metabolize stored body fat and tone up muscle tissue.

BEST NATURAL SOURCES:

Nuts, popcorn, carob, gelatin desserts, chocolate, brown rice, oatmeal, raisins, sunflower and sesame seeds, whole wheat bread, and all protein-rich foods.

SUPPLEMENT GUIDE:

L-arginine is available in tablets or powder. It's best taken on an empty stomach (with juice or water) in a 2-gram (2,000 mg.) dose immediately before retiring. Additional benefits — particularly those for muscle-toning — can be gained by taking 2 grams (2,000 mg.) on an empty stomach (with juice or water) one hour prior to engaging in vigorous physical exercise.
CAUTIONS: Do not give to growing children (could cause giantism) or persons with schizophrenic conditions.

Arginine supplements — and arginine-rich foods — are contraindicated for anyone who has herpes.

Dosages exceeding 20–30 grams daily are not recommended. They could cause enlarged joints and deformities of bones.

103

Arginine is necessary for adults because after the age of 30 there is almost a complete cessation of its secretion from the pituitary gland.

If you notice a thickening or coarsening of your skin, you're taking too much arginine. Several weeks of extremely high doses can cause this side effect, but it is reversible. Just cut back on your intake.

Any physical trauma increases your need for dietary arginine.

L-arginine taken in conjunction with L-ornithine can help stimulate weight loss.

Growth Hormone (G.H.) Releasers

Growth Hormone (G.H.) Releasers are nutrients that stimulate the production of growth hormone in the body. The human Growth Hormone is stored in the pituitary gland and the body releases it in response to sleep, exercise, and restricted food intake.

WHAT GROWTH HORMONE CAN DO FOR YOU:

Help burn fat and convert it into energy and muscle.

Improve resistance to disease.

Accelerate wound-healing.

Aid in tissue repair.

Strengthen connective tissue for healthier tendons and ligaments.

Enhance protein synthesis for muscle growth.

Reduce urea levels in blood and urine.

Important G.H. Releasers are the amino acids ornithine, arginine, tryptophan, glycine, and tyrosine, which work synergistically (more effectively together than separately) with vitamin B_6, niacinamide, zinc, calcium, magnesium, potassium, and vitamin C to trigger the night-time release of growth hormone. Peak secretion of G.H. is reached about 90 minutes after we fall asleep.

Natural growth hormone levels decrease as we grow older. Somewhere around age 50, G.H. production virtually stops completely. But by supplementing your diet with the amino acids and vitamins that stimulate release of growth hormone, production can be brought back up to the levels of a young adult.

THE DYNAMIC AMINO DUO: ORNITHINE & ARGININE

Ornithine and arginine, two of the amino acids involved in the release of human growth hormone, are among the most popular amino acid supplements today, essentially because they can help you slim down and shape up while you sleep (which is when G.H. is secreted). While some hormones encourage the body to store fat, growth hormone acts as a mobilizer of fat, helping you to not only look trimmer but have more energy as well.

Ornithine stimulates insulin secretion and helps insulin work as an anabolic (muscle-building) hormone, which has increased its use among body builders. Taking extra ornithine will help increase the levels of arginine in your body. (Actually, arginine is constructed from ornithine and ornithine is released from arginine in a continuing cyclic process.)

Because ornithine and arginine are so closely related, the characteristics and cautions for one apply to the other. (See section on "Arginine.") As a supplement, ornithine works best when taken at the same time and in the same manner as arginine (on an empty stomach, with juice or water — no protein).

Other Amino Acids

GLUTAMINE & GLUTAMIC ACID

Glutamic acid serves primarily as a brain fuel. It has the ability to pick up excess ammonia — which can inhibit high-performance brain function — and convert it into the buffer glutamine. Since glutamine produces marked elevation of glutamic acid, a shortage of the former in the diet can result in a shortage of the latter in the brain.

Aside from improving intelligence (even the IQs of mentally deficient children), glutamine has been shown to help in the control of alcoholism. It has also been found to shorten the healing time for ulcers and alleviate fatigue, depression, and impotence. Most recently it's been used successfully in the treatment of schizophrenia and senility.

L-glutamine (the natural form of glutamine) is available as a

105

supplement in 500 mg. capsules. The recommended dosage is 1–4 grams (1,000–4,000 mg.) daily, in divided doses. (For fatigue, depression, and impotence, the recommended dosage is 500 to 1,000 mg. daily for the first few weeks, 1,200–1,500 mg. for the next few weeks, and finally 2,000 mg. after a month.)

ASPARTIC ACID

Aspartic acid aids in the expulsion of harmful ammonia from the body. When ammonia enters the circulatory system, it acts as a highly toxic substance. By disposing of ammonia, aspartic acid helps protect the central nervous system. Recent research indicates that it may be an important factor in increased resistance to fatigue. When salts of aspartic acid were given to athletes, they showed decidedly improved stamina and endurance.

L-aspartic acid (the natural form of aspartic acid) is available as a supplement in 250 mg. and 500 mg. tablets. The usual dosage is 500 mg. 1–3 times daily with juice or water (no protein).

CYSTINE & CYSTEINE

Cystine is the *stable form* of the sulphur-containing amino acid cysteine (an important anti-aging nutrient). The body readily converts one into the other as needed, and the two forms can be considered as a single amino acid in metabolism. When cystine is metabolized, it yields sulphuric acid, which reacts with other substances to help detoxify the system.

Sulphur-containing amino acids, particularly cystine and methionine, have been shown to be effective protectors against copper toxicity. An excessive accumulation of copper in humans is a sign of Wilson's disease. Cystine/cysteine can also help "tie up" and protect the body from other harmful metals as well as destructive free radicals that are formed by smoking and drinking. A cysteine supplement (L-cystine) taken daily with vitamin C (three times as much vitamin C as cysteine) is the regimen that's been suggested for smokers and alcohol drinkers. Supplements need not be taken on an empty stomach. Recent research also indicates that therapeutic doses of cysteine can offer an important degree of protection against X-ray and nuclear radiation.

CAUTION: Large doses of cysteine/cystine, vitamins C and B_1 are not recommended for anyone with diabetes mellitus, and should only be undertaken on the advice of a physician. (The combination of these nutrients could negate insulin effectiveness.)

METHIONINE

Like cystine, this is another sulphur-containing amino acid. Methionine helps in some cases of schizophrenia by lowering the blood level of histamine, which can cause the brain to relay wrong messages. When combined with choline and folic acid, it has been shown to offer protection against certain tumours.

An insufficiency of methionine can break down the body's ability to process urine and result in oedema (swelling due to retention of fluids in tissues) and susceptibility to infection. A methionine deficiency has also been linked to cholesterol deposits, atherosclerosis, and hair loss in laboratory animals.

GLYCINE

Sometimes referred to as the simplest of the amino acids, glycine has been shown to yield quite a few remarkable benefits. It has been found helpful in the treatment of low pituitary gland function, and, because it supplies the body with additional creatine (essential for muscle function), it has also been found effective in the treatment of progressive muscular dystrophy.

Many nutritionally oriented doctors now use glycine in the treatment of hypoglycaemia. (Glycine stimulates the release of glucagon, which mobilizes glycogen, which is then released into the blood as glucose.)

Additionally, it is effective as a treatment for gastric hyperacidity (and is included in many gastric antacid drugs). It has also been used to treat certain types of acidaemia (low pH of the blood), especially one caused by a leucine imbalance which results in an offensive body and breath odour (a condition formerly treated only by a dietary restriction of leucine).

TYROSINE

Though this is a nonessential amino acid, it's a high-ranking neuro-transmitter, and important because of its role in stimulating and modifying brain activity. For instance, in order for phenylalanine to be effective as a mood elevator, appetite depressant, etc., it must first convert into tyrosine. If this conversion does not take place, either because of some enzyme insufficiency or a great need elsewhere in the body for phenylalanine, insufficient quantities of noradrenaline will be produced by the brain and depression will result.

Clinical studies have shown that tyrosine supplementation has helped control medication-resistant depression and anxiety, as well as enable patients taking amphetamines (as mood elevators or diet drugs) to reduce their dosages to minimal levels in a matter of weeks.

Tyrosine has also helped cocaine addicts conquer their habit by helping to avert the depression, fatigue, and extreme irritability which accompany withdrawal. A regimen of tyrosine, dissolved in orange juice, taken along with vitamin C, tyrosine hydroxylase (the enzyme that lets the body use tyrosine), and vitamins B_1, B_2, and niacin seems to work.

Any Questions About Chapter VI?

I'm prone to convulsions, and my doctor put me on phenytoin a year ago. Recently, a friend told me about Taurine, which she said was a nonessential amino acid that was natural and could help me in the same way. What I want to know is, if it's nonessential why would I need it? And why would it work?

Let me begin by clearing up a major point of misunderstanding: where amino acids are concerned, nonessential does *not* mean unnecessary. All the amino acids are necessary, it's just that the ones that are deemed essential can't be synthesized by the body in sufficient quantities to promote effective protein synthesis. If these essential ones are not supplied in the diet, *all* amino acids are reduced in the same proportion as the one that's low or missing. As for substituting Taurine for an anticonvulsant medication, that's a decision only your doctor can make. I can say though that Taurine has been shown to be quite successful as an anti-convulsant when taken in combination with glutamic and aspartic acids, but would not recommend undertaking it without consulting a doctor.

I've read that exercise stimulates the release of growth hormone. I do at least twenty minutes of dance exercise every day, so does this mean that I probably don't need a G.H. supplement?

On the contrary, you probably do. Only certain exercises, such as weight-lifting, where there is what's known as muscular "peak output" (even briefly sustained), promote a significant release of G.H. Other exercises, even prolonged ones, produce negligible amounts (if any) of growth hormone — unless they are performed with peak muscular effort. In fact, because amino acids are lost through the skin when you sweat, exercise *increases* your need for amino acids that will stimulate growth hormone.

I take a well-known patent slimming tablet to control my weight. On the label it says that it contains phenylpropanolamine. Is this the same as L-phenylalanine, and are they equally effective?

Phenylpropanolamine (PPA), which is found in many diet pills, is definitely *not* the same as L-phenylalanine. PPA is an appetite depressant (of dubious effectiveness, according to the American Medical Association) with a high incidence of side effects, including adverse interactions with MAO inhibitors and some oral contraceptives. Unlike the amino acid phenylalanine, which stimulates the brain to produce noradrenaline (which has been shown to reduce hunger) and alleviate those down-in-the-dumps diet blues, PPA depletes the brain of noradrenaline – usually in about two weeks — and leaves dieters fatigued and often depressed.

PPA is a poor substitute for a good diet while L-phenylalanine, which is found naturally in such protein-rich foods as cottage cheese, soy products, almonds, dry skim milk, and many more, can aid in appetite control (while nourishing the brain) if taken one hour before meals with juice or water.

Is there such a thing as an anti-aging amino acid?

As a matter of fact, L-glutathione (GSH) has been called a triple threat anti-aging amino acid. It's actually a tripeptide, synthesized from three amino acids — L-cysteine, L-glutamic acid, and glycine, and it has been shown to act as an antioxidant and deactivate free radicals which speed up the aging process. It

109

is also an anti-tumour agent, a respiratory accelerator in the brain, and has been used to help in the treatment of allergies, cataracts, diabetes, hypoglycaemia, and arthritis, as well as in helping to prevent the harmful side effects of high-dose radiation in chemotherapy and X-rays. Additionally, it helps to protect against the harmful effects of cigarette smoke and alcohol.

What is this new amino acid L-carnitine that I have been hearing about?

We're all very excited about it, since recent research has indicated that not only does it play an important role in converting stored body fat into energy, but it can help control hypoglycaemia, reduce angina attacks, and benefit patients with diabetes, liver or kidney disease.

The heart is dependent upon L-carnitine, and a deficiency of this amino acid can cause impairment of heart tissue. The major natural sources are meats and dairy products.

With diseases such as cancer, AIDS, and what have you on the rampage these days, is there anything that can be done to improve an individual's immune system?

Fortunately, yes! The answer seems to be Growth Hormone Releasers.

What happens is that as we get older, our immune system — that ever-ready army of white blood cells (called T-cells because they're under the command of the thymus gland) which are told where and when to attack and what antibodies their cofighters (called B-cells because they're made in the bone marrow) should produce — begins to break down due to the decreasing power and size of the thymus gland. This not only causes an ineffectual defense system, but often dangerous confusion where the T-cells mistake friends for enemies and attack you, resulting in autoimmune disorders. It's been suggested that diseases such as multiple sclerosis, myasthenia gravis, and arthritis may be due to this.

What's been discovered recently, though, is that this is most likely due to a reduced rate of growth hormone, which is produced by the pituitary gland and necessary to the function of the thymus gland and therefore the immune system. But supplements of amino acids (arginine, ornithine, and cysteine), as well as vitamins E, A, C, zinc, selenium, and enzymes such as papain, have been found to work wonders in reversing this degenerative syndrome.

VII

Other Wonder Workers

Acidophilus

Lactobacilus acidophilus, or acidophilus, as it is commonly known, is a source of friendly intestinal bacteria and more effective than yoghurt. It is available as acidophilus culture, incubated in soya, milk, or yeast bases.

Many doctors prescribe acidophilus in conjunction with oral antibiotic treatment because antibiotics destroy beneficial intestinal flora, often causing diarrhoea as well as an overgrowth of the fungus, monilia abricans. This fungus can grow in the intestines, vagina, lungs, mouth [thrush], on the fingers, or under the nails. It will usually disappear after a few days use of general amounts of acidophilus culture.

Regular use of acidophilus culture keeps the intestines clean. It can eliminate bad breath caused by intestinal putrefaction [the sort resistant to mouthwash or breath spray], constipation, foul-smelling flatulence, and aid in the treatment of acne and other skin problems.

Keep in mind that lactose, complex carbohydrates, pectin, and vitamin C plus roughage encourage additional growth of intestinal flora. This is important since friendly bacteria can die within five days unless they are continuously supplied with some form of lactic acid or lactose — like acidophilus.

111

Ginseng

It is generally well accepted that ginseng is a stimulant of both mental and physical energy. The Chinese have been using it for nearly five thousand years and still revere it as a preventive and cure-all. It is a mild laxative and helps the body pass poisons through more rapidly. Its reputed benefits include cures for impotence, high and low blood pressure, anaemia, arthritis, indigestion, insomnia, fatigue, hypoglycaemia, poor circulation, and more.

Miracles aside, ginseng does help you assimilate vitamins and minerals by acting as an endocrine-gland stimulant. It is best to take it on an empty stomach, preferably before breakfast, if you want it to be its most effective.

Vitamin C has been said to neutralise part of ginseng's value, but there is no real evidence to support this. [If you take a vitamin-C supplement, the time-release form makes any counteraction less likely].

Ginseng is available in capsule form; It can also be purchased as tea, liquid concentrate, or as ginseng root in a bottle.

Alfalfa, Garlic, Chlorophyll, and Yucca

Alfalfa has been dubbed "the great healer" by noted biologist and author Frank Bouer, who discovered that the green leaves of this remarkable legume contain *eight* essential enzymes. Also, for every 100 g., it contains 8,000 IU of vitamin A and 20,000 to 40,000 units of vitamin K, which protects against haemorrhaging and helps in blood clotting. It is additionally a fine source of vitamins B_6 and E, and contains enough vitamin D, lime, and phosphorus to secure strong bones and teeth in growing children.

Many doctors have used alfalfa in treating stomach ailments, gas pains, ulcerous conditions, and poor appetite because it contains vitamin U, which is also found in raw cabbage and cabbage juice. The latter has frequently been used as an aid in treating peptic ulcers. Alfalfa is also a good laxative and a natural diuretic.

Garlic contains potassium, phosphorus, a significant amount of B and C vitamins, as well as calcium and protein.

112

It does appear to have some amazing properties. Many medical authorities feel that it can reduce high blood pressure by either neutralising the poisonous substances in the intestines or acting as a vasodilator. F.G. Piotrousky, of the University of Vienna, found that 40 percent of his hypertensive patients had substantially lower blood pressure after they were given garlic.

Garlic has also been found to be effective in cleansing the blood of excess glucose. [Blood sugar ranks with cholesterol as a causitive factor in arteriosclerosis and heart attacks.] In addition, it has also been reported to alleviate grippe, sore throat, and bronchial congestion.

The best way to take garlic as a supplement is in the form of perles. These caps contain the valuable garlic oils and leave no after-odour on the breath, because they do not dissolve in the stomach but in the lower digestive tract. Garlic tablets with parsley [which contains natural chlorophyll] are also available.

Chlorophyll, according to G.W. Rapp in the *American Journal of Pharmacy*, possesses positive antibacterial action. It also appears to act as a wound-healing agent, and while stimulating the growth of new tissue, it reduces the hazard of bacterial contamination.

Nature's deodorant, it is used in commercial air fresheners, as a topical body deodorant and as an oral breath refresher. It is available in tablets and in liquid preparations.

Yucca extract comes from the genus of trees and shrubs belonging to the Liliaceae family. [The Joshua tree is a yucca.] The Indians used the yucca for many purposes and revered it as a plant that guaranteed their health and survival. Dr. John W. Yale, a botanical biochemist, extracted the steroid saponin from the plant and used the extract in a tablet for the treatment of arthritis. The treatment proved safe and effective, the average dose being four tablets daily, and there was no gastrointestinal irritation. Yucca-extract tablets are nontoxic and available in most health-food and vitamin stores.

Bran and Fibre

Recent research indicates that we would all be a great deal

healthier and live longer if we ate coarser diets that sent more indigestible dietary fibre through our digestive tracts.

The best way to increase your fibre intake is to eat breads made of 100 percent whole grains, raw fruit, and to add unprocessed bran to your daily diet [it can be mixed into your regular breakfast cereal]. Bran has little or no food value. We do not digest and absorb it. As it passes through the digestive tract, it accumulates liquid and swells up, providing a good amount of soft bulk that speeds bowel movements and acts to dilute levels of fat metabolites associated with carcinogen formation. Bran is also available as a food supplement in concentrated tablet form.

When research appeared indicating that we would all be a great deal healthier and live longer if we ate coarser diets that sent more indigestible dietary fibre through our digestive tracts, a lot of people, wisely, jumped on the fibre bandwagon, though most weren't aware (and still aren't) that all fibre is not the same and that different types perform different functions.

TYPES OF FIBRE YOU SHOULD KNOW ABOUT

Cellulose This is found in whole-wheat flour, bran, cabbage, young peas, green beans, wax beans, broccoli, brussels sprouts, cucumber skins, peppers, apples, and carrots.

Hemicelluloses These are found in bran, cereals, whole grains, brussels sprouts, mustard greens, and beet root.

Cellulose and hemicelluloses absorb water and can smooth functioning of the large bowel. Essentially, they "bulk" waste and move it through the colon more rapidly. This not only can prevent constipation, but may also protect against diverticulosis, spastic colon, hemorrhoids, cancer of the colon, and varicose veins.

Gums These are usually found in oatmeal and other rolled oat products as well as in dried beans.

Pectin This is found in apples, citrus fruits, carrots, cauliflower, cabbage, dried peas, green beans, potatoes, squash, and strawberries.

Gums and pectin primarily influence absorption in the stomach and small bowel. By binding with bile acids, they decrease fat absorption and lower cholesterol levels. They delay stomach-

emptying by coating the lining of the gut, and by so doing they slow sugar absorption after a meal, which is helpful to diabetics since it reduces the amount of insulin needed at any one time.

Lignin This type of fibre is found in breakfast cereals, bran, older vegetables (when vegetables age, their lignin content rises, and they become less digestible), aubergine, green beans, strawberries, pears, and radishes.

Lignin reduces the digestibility of other fibres. It also binds with bile acids to lower cholesterol and helps speed food through the gut.

CAUTION: While it's true that most of us still don't have enough fibre in our diet, too much can cause gas, bloating, nausea, vomiting, diarrhoea, and possibly interfere with your body's ability to absorb certain minerals, such as zinc, calcium, iron, magnesium, as well as vitamin B_{12}, though this is easily prevented by varying your diet along with your high-fibre foods.

Kelp

This amazing seaweed contains more vitamins and minerals than any other food. To be more specific, kelp has vitamin B_2, niacin, choline, carotene, and algenic acid, as well as twenty-three minerals which range as follows:

Iodine	0.15–0.20%	Magnesium	0.70%
Calcium	1.20%	Sulphur	0.93%
Phosphorus	0.30%	Chlorine	12.21%
Iron	0.10%	Copper	0.0008%
Sodium	3.14%	Zinc	0.0003%
Potassium	0.63%	Manganese	0.0008%

Plus traces of: barium, boron, chromium, lithium, nickel, silver, titanium, vanadium, aluminium, strontium, and silicon. Because of its natural iodine content, kelp has a normalising effect on the thyroid gland. In other words, thin people with thyroid trouble can gain weight by using kelp and obese people can lose weight with it.

Homeopathic physicians use kelp for obesity, poor digestion, flatulence, and obstinate constipation; and, for the past several years, one of the most widespread fads has been the kelp, lecithin, vinegar, and B_6 diet.

115

Yeast

One of the richest sources of organic iron. It's known as nature's wonder food, and it does a lot to deserve its reputation. Yeast is an excellent source of protein and a superior source of the natural B-complex vitamins. It is one of the richest sources of organic iron and a gold mine of minerals, trace minerals, and amino acids. It has been known to help lower cholesterol [when combined with lecithin], help reverse gout, and ease the aches and pains of neuritis.

There are various sources of yeast:

Brewer's yeast [from hops, a by-product of beer], sometimes called nutritional yeast.
Torula yeast grown on wood pulp used in the manufacture of paper. Or from blackstrap molasses.
Whey, a by-product of milk and cheese [best-tasting and most potent].
Liquid yeast frim Switzerland and Germany, fed on herbs, honey malt, and oranges or grapefruit.

Avoid live baker's yeast! Live cells deplete the B vitamins in the intestines and rob your body of all vitamins. In nutritional yeast, these live cells are heat-killed, thus preventing that depletion.

Yeast has all the major B vitamins [except B_{12}], which can be especially bred into it. It contains sixteen amino acids, fourteen or more minerals, and seventeen vitamins [except for A, E and C]. It can be considered a whole food.

Because yeast, like other protein foods, is high in phosphorus, it is advisable when taking it to add extra calcium to the diet. Phosphorus, though a co-worker of calcium, can take calcium out of the body, leaving a deficiency. The remedy is simple: increase your calcium [calcium lactate assimilates well in the body]. *B-complex vitamins should be taken together with yeast to be more effective. Together they work like a powerhouse.*

Yeast can be stirred into liquid, juice, or water and taken between meals. Many people who feel fatigued take a tablespoon or more in liquid and feel a return of energy within minutes, and the good effects last for several hours. Yeast can also be used as a reducing food. Stir into liquid and drink just before a meal. It takes the edge off a large appetite and saves you a lot in calories.

VIII

How to Find Out What Vitamins You Really Need

What Is a Balanced Diet and Are You Eating It?

A balanced diet is something easily found in books and rarely on the table. Though nutrients are widely scattered all through our food supply, soil depletion, storage, food processing, and cooking destroy many of them. Still, there are enough left to make balancing meals important. After all, supplements cannot work without food, and the better the food you eat, the more effective your supplements will be. Unfortunately, no possible "balanced" diet is likely to meet nutritional needs today.

Nevertheless, to know whether or not you are balancing your meals, you should become familiar with the four basic food groups, and the recommended number of portions that should be eaten from them each day. Serving sizes should be individually determined; smaller amounts for less active people, larger amounts for teenagers and people who do physically strenuous work.

MILK GROUP

Milk, cheese, yoghurt, foods made from milk.

> 3 servings per day for a child
> 4 servings per day for a teenager
> 2 servings per day for an adult
> 4 servings per day for pregnant and lactating women

MEAT GROUP

Beef, veal, pork, lamb, fish, poultry, liver, or eggs. Dry peas, beans, soya extenders, and nuts combined with animal protein — including eggs, milk, and cheese — or grain protein can be substituted for meat servings.

117

2 servings per day
3 servings per day for pregnant women

FRUIT-VEGETABLE GROUP

Citrus or other fruit rich in vitamin C [or tomato juice] should be eaten daily. Dark-green, leafy, or orange vegetables and fruit should be eaten three or four times a week for vitamin A.

4 servings per day

GRAIN GROUP

Whole or enriched grains, bread in any shape, hot or cold cereals, macaroni, noodles, or other pasta.

4 servings per day

The recommended servings, as outlined by the National Research Council, are designed to supply 1,200 calories. You are expected to adjust the size of the servings to suit your own individual growth, weight, and energy needs.

How to Test for Deficiencies

If you're wondering whether or not you need vitamin or mineral supplementation, your best bet would be to contact a nutritionally orientated doctor. Other than that, there are a variety of "indicator" tests that should tell you enough to point you in the right supplement direction.

Dr. John M. Ellis has devised a quick early-warning test for B_6 [pyridoxine] deficiency. Extend your hand, palm up, then try to bend the two joints in your four fingers [not the knuckles of your hand] until your fingertips reach your palm. [This is not a fist, only two joints are bent.] Do this with both hands. If it is difficult, if finger joints don't allow tips to reach your palm, a pyridoxine deficiency is likely.

Betty Lee Morales, a well-known nutritionist, says that urine is a fair indicator of the B vitamins in your body. Since B vitamins are water soluble and lost each day through excretion, when your body demands more your urine will be light in colour. When the urine is dark, your B demands are less. [*Note:* Many drugs, illnesses, and foods also alter urine colour. This should be taken into consideration.]

Possible Warning Signs

A body in need of vitamins usually lets you know about it sooner or later. It's unlikely that any of us will come down with scurvy before realising we need vitamin C, but more often than not our bodies are giving us clues that we just don't recognise. With the price of medical insurance rising daily, paying attention to your nutritional warning system is about the best and cheapest insurance around. Here are a few common *symptoms* that you might be ignoring — and shouldn't.

The supplements recommended are not intended as medical advice, only as a guide in working with your doctor.

POSSIBLE DEFICIENCY	ARE YOU EATING ENOUGH?	RECOMMENDED SUPPLEMENT
	Appetite Loss	
Protein	Meat, fish, eggs, dairy products, soya beans, peanuts	1 B complex, 50 mg., taken with each meal. 1 B_{12}, 2,000 mcg. [time
Vitamin A	Fish, liver, egg yolks, butter, cream, green leafy or yellow vegetables	release] with breakfast. 1 organic iron complex tablet [containing vitamin C, copper, liver,
Vitamin B_1	Brewer's yeast, whole grains, meat [pork or liver], nuts, legumes, potatoes	manganese, and zinc] to help assimilate
Vitamin C	Citrus fruits, tomatoes, potatoes, cabbage, green peppers	

[*Note:* NSP stands for Nutrition Starter Package. This consists of a high-potency multiple vitamin with chelated minerals, preferably time release; a vitamin C, 1,000 mg. with bioflavonoids, rutin, hesperidin, and rose hips, time release; a high-potency chelated multiple-mineral supplement. One of each to be taken with breakfast and dinner.]

119

POSSIBLE DEFICIENCY	ARE YOU EATING ENOUGH?	RECOMMENDED SUPPLEMENT
Appetite Loss		
Biotin	Brewer's yeast, nuts, beef liver, kidney, unpolished rice	
Phosphorus	Milk, cheese, meat, poultry, fish, cereals, nuts, legumes	
Sodium	Beef, pork, sardines, cheese, green olives, corn bread, sauerkraut	
Zinc	Vegetables, whole grains, wheat bran, wheat germ, pumpkin seeds, sunflower seeds	
Bad Breath		
Niacin	Liver, meat, fish, whole whole grains, legumes	1–2 tbsp. acidiphilus liquid [flavoured] 1 to 3 times a day. 1 chlorophyll tablet or capsule 3 times a day. 1–3 chelated zinc 50-mg. tabs 3 times a day. 1–2 multiple digestive enzyme tabs 1–3 times a day
Body Odour		
B_{12}	Yeast, liver, beef, eggs, kidney	Same as bad breath
*Bruising Easily**		
Vitamin C	Citrus fruits, tomatoes, potatoes, cabbage, green peppers	1 C complex, 1,000 mg. [time release] with bioflavonoids, rutin and hesperidin A.M. and P.M.
Bioflavonoids	Orange, lemon, lime, tangerine peels	

* When slight or minor injuries produce bluish, purplish discolouration of skin.

POSSIBLE DEFICIENCY	ARE YOU EATING ENOUGH?	RECOMMENDED SUPPLEMENT
High Cholesterol		
B complex Inositol	Yeast, brewer's yeast, dried lima beans, raisins, cantaloupe	1 tbsp, acidophilus liquid 3 times daily or 3 caps 3 times daily. 2–3 tbsp. lecithin granules 3–4 times daily [used on salads or cottage cheese] or 3 1,200-mg. caps 3–4 times daily.
Constipation		
B complex	Liver, beef, cheese, pork, kidney	1 tbsp. acidophilus liquid 3 times daily. 3–9 bran tabs daily.
Diarrhoea		
Vitamin K Niacin Vitamin F	Yoghurt, alfalfa, soyabean oil, fish, liver, oils, kelp Liver, lean meat, brewer's yeast, peanuts, dried nutritional yeast, white meat of poultry, avocado, fish, legumes, whole grain Vegetable oils, peanuts, sunflower seeds, walnuts	1 g. potassium divided over 3 meals. As a preventive 1–2 tbsp. acidophilus liquid [flavoured] 3 times daily
Dizziness		
Manganese	Nuts, green leafy vegetables, peas, beets, egg yolks	50–100 mg. niacin 3 times a day. 400 IU vitamin E
Diarrhoea		
B_2 [Riboflavin]	Milk, liver, kidney, yeast, cheese, fish, eggs	1–3 times a day

POSSIBLE DEFICIENCY	ARE YOU EATING ENOUGH?	RECOMMENDED SUPPLEMENT
	Ear Noises	
Manganese	See above	Same as for dizziness
Potassium	Bananas, watercress, all leafy greeen vegetables, citrus fruits, sunflower seeds	
	Eye Problems*	
Vitamin A	See above	10,000 IU vitamin A
B$_2$ [Riboflavin]	See above	1–3 times daily for 5 days and stop for 2. 100 mg. B complex [time release], 1 in A.M. and P.M. 500 mg. vitamin C with bioflavonoids, rutin, and hesperidin, 1 in A.M. and P.M. 400 IU vitamin E [dry], 1 in A.M. and P.M.

* Night blindness, inability to adjust to darkness, bloodshot eyes, inflammation, burning sensations, styes.

	Fatigue*	
Zinc	Vegetables, wholegrain products, brewer's yeast, wheat bran, wheat germ, pumpkin and sunflower seeds	1 B complex, 100 mg. [time release] 2 times, daily. 1 2,000-mcg. B$_{12}$ A.M. and P.M. 1 50-mg. B$_{15}$ with each meal, NSP, 1 A.M. and P.M.
Carbohydrates	Cellulose	
Protein	See above	
Vitamin A	See above	
Vitamin B complex	See above	
PABA	Same as B complex	
Iron	Wheat germ, Soyabean flour, beef, kidney, liver, beans, clams, peaches and molasses	
Iodine	Seafoods, dairy products, kelp	
Vitamin C	See above	
Vitamin D	Fish liver oils, butter, egg yolk, liver, sunshine	

* Lassitude, weakness, no inclination for physical activity.

POSSIBLE DEFICIENCY	ARE YOU EATING ENOUGH?	RECOMMENDED SUPPLEMENT
*Gastrointestinal Problems**		
Vitamin B₁ [thiamin]	See above	25,000 IU vitamin A 1–3 times daily. Take for
Vitamin B₂ [riboflavin]	See above	5 days and stop for 2
Folic acid [folacin]	Fresh green leafy vegetables, fruit, organ meats, liver, dried nutritional yeast	100 mg. B complex [time release], 1 A.M. and P.M. Multiple minerals, 1 A.M. and P.M.
PABA	Same as B complex; see above	
Vitamin C	See above	
Chlorine	Kelp, rye flour, ripe olives, sea greens	
Pantothenic acid	Same as B complex; see above	

* Gastritis, gastric ulcers, gallbladder, digestive disturbances.

Hair Problems

1. DANDRUFF*

Vitamin B₁₂ [cyanocobalamin]	Liver, beef, pork, organ meats, eggs, milk and milk products	50 mcg. selenium 3 times daily. NSP, 1 A.M. and P.M.
Vitamin F	See above	
Vitamin B₆	Dried nutritional yeast, liver, organ meats, legumes, whole-grain cereals, fish	
Selenium	Bran, germ of cereals, broccoli, onions, tomatoes, and tuna	

* Loose flakes – dry or yellow and greasy – which fall from scalp.

2. DULL, DRY, BRITTLE, OR GREYING HAIR

Vitamin B complex	See above	3 vitamin-F caps with each meal. 3–6 lecithin caps with each meal NSP, 1 A.M. and P.M.
PABA	Same as B complex see above	
Vitamin F	See above	
Iodine	Seafoods, iodised salt, dairy products	

POSSIBLE DEFICIENCY	ARE YOU EATING ENOUGH?	RECOMMENDED SUPPLEMENT
	3. LOSS OF HAIR	
Biotin	See above	Stress B, 600 mg., 2
Inositol	Unrefined molasses and liver, lecithin, unprocessed whole grains, citrus fruits, brewer's yeast	times daily. 1,000 mg. choline and inositol daily. 1 multiple mineral daily
Chlorine	Sodium chloride [table salt]	
B complex with C and folic acid	See above	

Heart Palpitation

Vitamin B$_{12}$ [cobalamin, cyanocobalamin]	See above mg. vitamin B complex [time release] A.M. and	NSP, 1 A.M. and P.M. 100
		P.M. 100 mg. niacin 1–3 times daily. 3 caps lecithin 3 times daily

High Blood Pressure

Choline	Egg yolks, brain, heart, green leafy vegetables, yeast, liver, wheat germ	Lecithin granules, 3 tbsp. daily or 3 caps 3 times daily. NSP, 1 A.M. and P.M. Start with 100 IU vitamin E and work up to higher strengths. 1–3 kelp tabs daily. 1 garlic perle 3 times daily

Infections (high susceptibility)

Vitamin A (carotene)	Fish, liver, egg yolks, butter, cream, green leafy or yellow vegetables	1–2 tbsp. acidophilus 3 times daily. Vitamin A up to 10,000 IU every other day for duration of infection. 1 NSP A.M.
Pantothenic acid	Yeast, brewer's yeast, dried lima beans, raisins, cantaloupe	and P.M. (2–5 g. vitamin C for duration of infection)

124

POSSIBLE DEFICIENCY	ARE YOU EATING ENOUGH?	RECOMMENDED SUPPLEMENT
	Insomnia	
Potassium	Bananas, watercress, all leafy green vegetables, citrus fruits, sunflower seeds	2 g. tryptophan ½ hr. before bedtime. Vitamin B_6 100 mg., niacinamide 100 mg., and chelated
B complex	Yeast, brewer's yeast, dried lima beans, raisins, cantaloupe	calcium and magnesium ½ hr. before bedtime. 1 NSP A.M. and P.M.
Biotin	Brewer's yeast, nuts, beef liver, kidney, unpolished rice	
Calcium	Milk and milk products, meat, fish, eggs, cereal products, beans, fruit, vegetables	
	Loss of smell	
Vitamin A	See above	50 mg. chelated zinc 3
Zinc	See above	times daily [cut back to 1–2 daily when condition improves]
	Memory Loss	
B_1 [thiamine]	See above	L-glutamine, 500 mg. 3 times daily. 50 mg. B complex A.M. and P.M. Choline, 2g. daily in divided doses
	Menstrual Problems	
B_{12}	Yeast, liver, beef, eggs, kidney	7–10 days before period: 1 NSP A.M. and P.M. 100 mg. B_6 3 times daily. 100 mg. B complex [time release] A.M. and P.M. Evening Primrose oil, 500 mg. 3 times daily. 500 mg. magnesium and ½ as much calcium once daily

POSSIBLE DEFICIENCY	ARE YOU EATING ENOUGH?	RECOMMENDED SUPPLEMENT
Mouth Sores and Cracks		
Vitamin B_2 [riboflavin]	Milk, liver, kidney, yeast, cheese, fish, eggs	50 mg. B complex 3 times daily with meals. 1
Vitamin B_6 [pyridoxine]	Dried nutritional yeast, liver, organ meats, legumes, whole-grain cereals, fish	times daily with meals. 1 NSP A.M. and P.M.

Muscle Cramps (general muscle weakness, tenderness in calf, night cramps)

POSSIBLE DEFICIENCY	ARE YOU EATING ENOUGH?	RECOMMENDED SUPPLEMENT
Vitamin B_1 [thiamin]	Brewer's yeast, whole grains, meat [pork or liver], nuts, legumes, potatoes	400 IU vitamin E [dry] 3 times daily. Chelated calcium and magnesium, 3 tabs 3 times daily. 100 mg. niacin 3 times daily
Vitamin B_6 [pyridoxine]	Dried nutritional yeast, liver, organ meats, legumes, whole-grain cereals, fish	
Biotin	Brewer's yeast, nuts, beef liver, kidney, unpolished rice	
Chlorine	Socium chloride [table salt]	
Sodium	Beef, pork, sardines, cheese, green olives, corn bread, sauerkraut	
Vitamin D [calciferol]	Fish-liver oils, butter, egg yolks, liver, sunshine	

Nervousness

POSSIBLE DEFICIENCY	ARE YOU EATING ENOUGH?	RECOMMENDED SUPPLEMENT
Vitamin B_6 [pyridoxine]	Dried nutritional yeast, liver, organ meats, legumes, whole-grain cereals, fish	Stress B with C 1–3 times daily [50 mg. of all B vitamins]. 500–667 mg. tryptophan 3 times daily between meals
Vitamin B_{12} [cyanocobalamin]	Yeast, liver, beef, eggs, kidney	[with juice or water] and 3 tabs at bedtime. 3
Niacin [nicotinic acid, niacinamide]	Liver, meat, fish, whole grains, legumes	chelated calcium and magnesium tabs 3 times
PABA	Yeast, brewer's yeast, dried lima beans, raisins, cantaloupe	daily. 1 NSP A.M. and P.M.
Magnesium	Green leafy vegetables, nuts, cereals, grains, seafoods	

POSSIBLE DEFICIENCY	ARE YOU EATING ENOUGH?	RECOMMENDED SUPPLEMENT

Nosebleeds

POSSIBLE DEFICIENCY	ARE YOU EATING ENOUGH?	RECOMMENDED SUPPLEMENT
Vitamin C	Citrus fruits, tomatoes, potatoes, cabbage, green peppers	1,000 mg. vitamin C with 50 mg. rutin, hesperidin, and 500 mg.
Vitamin K	Yogurt, alfalfa, soybean oil, fish-liver oils, kelp,	bioflavonoids [time release] A.M. and P.M.
Bioflavonoids	Orange, lemon, lime, tangerine peels	

Retarded Growth

Fat	Meat, butter	1 NSP A.M. and P.M.
Protein	Meat, fish, eggs, dairy products, soybeans, peanuts	
Vitamin B$_2$ [riboflavin]	Milk, liver, kidney, yeast, cheese, fish, eggs	
Folic acid	Fresh green leafy vegetables, fruit, organ meats, liver, dried nutritional yeast	
Zinc	Vegetables, whole grains, wheat bran, wheat germ, pumpkin and sunflower seeds	
Cobalt	Liver, kidney, pancreas, and spleen [organ meats]	

Skin Problems

1. ACNE (face blemishes, thickened skin, blackheads, whiteheads, red spots)

Water-solubilized vitamin A	Fish, liver, egg yolks, butter, cream, green leafy or yellow vegetables	1 multiple vitamin-mineral [low in iodine] daily. 1–2 400 IU vitamin E [dry] daily.
Vitamin B complex	Yeast, brewer's yeast, dried lima beans, raisins, cantaloupe	25,000 IU vitamin A [dry], 1–2 tabs daily 6 days a week. 50 mg. chelated zinc 3 times daily with food. 1–2 tbsp. acidophilus liquid 3 times daily or 3–6 caps 3 times daily. [Iodine worsens acne, so eliminate all processed foods – high in oidized salt – from your diet]

POSSIBLE DEFICIENCY	ARE YOU EATING ENOUGH?	RECOMMENDED SUPPLEMENT

2. DERMATITIS (skin inflammation)

POSSIBLE DEFICIENCY	ARE YOU EATING ENOUGH?	RECOMMENDED SUPPLEMENT
Vitamin B₂ [riboflavin]	Milk, liver, kidney, yeast, cheese, fish, eggs	1 multiple vitamin-mineral [low in iodine] daily. 1–2 400 IU vitamin E [dry] daily. 25,000 IU vitamin A [dry], 1–2 tabs daily 6 days a week. 50 mg. chelated zinc 3 times daily with food. 1–2 tbsp. acidophilus liquid 3 times daily or 3–6 caps 3 times daily
Vitamin B₆ [pyridoxine]	Dried nutritional yeast, liver, organ meats, legumes, whole-grain cereals, fish	
Biotin	Brewer's yeast, nuts, beef, liver, kidney, unpolished rice	
Niacin [nicotinic acid, niacinamide]	Liver, meat, fish, whole grains, legumes	

3. ECZEMA (rough, dry, scaly skin, redness and swelling, small blisters)

POSSIBLE DEFICIENCY	ARE YOU EATING ENOUGH?	RECOMMENDED SUPPLEMENT
Fat	Meat, butter	1 multiple vitamin-mineral [low in iodine] daily. 1–2 400 IU vitamin E [dry] daily. 25,000 IU vitamin A [dry], 1–2 tabs daily 6 days a week. 50 mg. chelated zinc 3 times daily with food. 1–2 tbsp. acidophilus liquid 3 times daily or 3–6 caps 3 times daily
Vitamin A [carotene]	Fish, liver, egg yolks, butter, cream, green leafy or yellow vegetables	
Vitamin B complex	Yeast, brewer's yeast, dried lima beans, raisins, cantaloupe	
Inositol		
Copper	Organ meats, oysters, nuts, dried legumes, whole-grain cereals	
Iodine	Seafoods, iodized salt, dairy products	

Slow-Healing Wounds and Fractures

POSSIBLE DEFICIENCY	ARE YOU EATING ENOUGH?	RECOMMENDED SUPPLEMENT
Vitamin C	Citrus fruits, tomatoes, potatoes, cabbage, green peppers	50 mg. zinc 3 times daily. 400 IU vitamin E 3 times daily. 1 NSP A.M. and P.M.

Softening of Bones and Teeth

POSSIBLE DEFICIENCY	ARE YOU EATING ENOUGH?	RECOMMENDED SUPPLEMENT
Vitamin D [calciferol]	Fish-liver oils, butter, egg yolks, liver, sunshine	1,000–1,500 mg. calcium, 500 mg. magnesium divided over 2 meals daily
Calcium	Milk and milk products, meat, fish, eggs cereal products, beans, fruit, vegetables	

POSSIBLE DEFICIENCY	ARE YOU EATING ENOUGH?	RECOMMENDED SUPPLEMENT
	Tremors	
Magnesium	Green leafy vegetables, nuts, cereals, grains, seafoods	B complex and 50 mg. B_6 3 times daily. 1,000 mg. calcium, 500 mg. magnesium divided over 3 meals daily
	Vaginal Itching	
Vitamin B_2	Milk, liver, kidney, yeast, cheese, fish, eggs	2 tbsp. acidophilus 3 times daily or 3–6 caps 3–4 times daily. (Acidophilus or vinegar douche can also help.)
	Water Retention	
Vitamin B_6	Dried nutritional yeast, liver, organ meats, legumes, whole-grain cereals, fish	100 mg. B_6 3 times daily
	White Spots on Nails	
Zinc	Vegetables, whole grains, wheat bran, wheat germ, pumpkin and sunflower seeds	50 mg. zinc 3 times daily. Stress B with C 1–2 times daily. 1 multiple mineral 2 times daily

Cravings — What They Might Mean

Cravings, which can sometimes mean allergies, are more often nature's way of letting you know that you're not getting enough of certain vitamins or minerals. Frequently these specific hungers develop because overall diet is inadequate.

Some of the most common cravings are:

Peanut Butter This is definitely among the top ten, and it's not at all surprising. Peanut butter is a rich source of B vitamins. If you find yourself dipping into the jar often, it might be because you're under stress and your ordinary B intake has become insufficient. Since 50 g. of peanut butter — a third of a cup — is 284 calories, you'll find it easier on your waistline to take a B-complex supplement if you do not want to gain weight.

Bananas When you catch yourself reaching for this fruit again and again, it could be because your body needs potassium. One medium banana has 555 mg. People taking diuretics or cortisone [which rob the body of needed potassium] often crave bananas.

Cheese If you're more a cheese luster than a cheese lover, there's a good chance that your real hunger is for calcium and phosphorus. [If it's processed cheese that you've been snacking on, you've been getting aluminium, too, without knowing it.] For one thing, you might try eating more broccoli. That's high in calcium and phosphorus, and a lot lower in calories than cheese.

Apples An apple a day doesn't necessarily keep the doctor away, but it offers a lot of good things that you might be missing in other foods — calcium, magnesium, phosphorus, potassium — and is an excellent source of cholesterol-lowering pectin! If you have a tendency to eat a lot of saturated fat, it could account for your apple cravings.

Butter Most often vegetarians crave butter because of their own low-saturated-fat intake, Salted butter, on the other hand, might be craved for the salt alone.

Cola The craving for cola is most often a sugar hunger and an addiction to caffeine. The beverage has no nutritive value.

Nuts If you're a little nutty about nuts, you probably could use more protein, B bitamins, or fat in your diet. If it's salted nuts you favour you could be craving the sodium and not the nuts. You'll find that people under stress tend to eat more nuts than relaxed individuals.

Ice cream High as ice cream is in calcium, most people crave it for its sugar content. Hypoglycaemics and diabetics have great hungers for it, as do people seeking to recapture the security of childhood.

Pickles If you're pregnant and want pickles, you're probably after the salt. And if you're not pregnant and crave pickles, the reason is most likely the same. [Pickles also contain a substantial amount of potassium.]

Bacon   Cravings for bacon are usually because of its fat. People on restricted diets are most susceptible to greasy binges. Unfortunately, saturated fat is not bacon's only drawback. Bacon is very high in carcinogenic nitrates. If you do indulge in bacon, be sure you're ingesting enough vitamin C and A, D and E to counteract the nitrates.

Eggs   Aside from the protein [two eggs give you 13 g.], sulphur, amino acids, and selenium, egg lovers might also be seeking the yolk's fat content or, paradoxically, its cholesterol- and fat-dissolving choline.

Cantaloupe   Just because you like its taste might not be the only reason you crave this melon. Cantaloupe is high in potassium and vitamin A. In fact, a quarter of a melon has 3,400 IU vitamin A. Since the melon also offers vitamin C, calcium, magnesium, phosphorus, biotin, and inositol, it's not a bad craving to give in to. There's only about 60 calories in half a melon.

Olives   Whether you crave them green or black, you're likely to be after the salt. People with underactive thyroids are most often the first to reach for them.

Salt   No guesswork here, it's the sodium you're after. Cravers quite possibly have a thyroid iodine deficiency or low sodium Addison's disease. Hypertensives often crave salt, and shouldn't.

Onions   Cravings for spicy foods can sometimes indicate problems in the lungs or sinuses.

Chocolate   Definitely one of the foremost cravings, if not *the* foremost. Chocoholics are addicted to the caffeine as well as the sugar. [There are 5 to 10 mg. of caffeine in a cup of cocoa.] If you want to kick the chocolate habit, try carob instead. [Carob, also called St. John's Bread, is made from the edible pods of the Mediterranean carob tree.]

Milk   If you're still craving milk as an adult, you might need a calcium supplement. Then again, it might be the amino acids — such as tryptophan, leucine, and lysine — that your body needs. Nervous people often seek out the tryptophan in milk, since it has a very soothing effect.

Chinese food   Of course it's delicious, but often it's the monosodium glutamate in the food that fosters the craving.

People with salt deficiencies usually go all out for Chinese food. [MSG can cause a histamine reaction in some individuals. Headaches and flushing may occur. Most Chinese restaurants will now prepare your food without MSG if you request it.]

Mayonnaise Since this is a fatty food, it is often craved by vegetarians and people who have eliminated other facts from their diet.

Tart fruits A persistent craving for tart fruits can often indicate problems with the gallbladder or liver.

Paint and dirt Children have a tendency to eat paint and dirt. Frequently this is an indication of a calcium or vitamin-D deficiency. A hard re-evaluation of your child's diet is essential, and a visit to your paediatrician is recommended.

Getting the Most Vitamins from Your Food

Eating the right foods doesn't necessarily mean that you're getting the vitamins they contain. Food processing, storing, and cooking can easily undermine the best nutritious intentions. To get the most from what you eat [not to mention what you spend] keep the following tips in mind:

Wash but don't soak fresh vegetables if you hope to benefit from the B vitamins and C they contain.

Forgo convenience and make your salads when you're ready to eat them. Fruits and vegetables cut up and left to stand lose vitamins.

If you don't plan to eat your fresh fruit or vegetables for a few days, you're better off buying fresh-frozen ones. The vitamin content of good frozen green beans will be higher than those fresh ones you've kept in your refrigerator for a week.

Don't thaw your frozen vegetables before cooking.

There are more vitamins in converted and parboiled rice than in polished rice, and brown rice is more nutritious than white.

Frozen foods that you can boil in their bags, offer more vitamins than the ordinary kind, and all frozen foods are preferable to canned ones.

Cooking in copper pots can destroy vitamin C, folic acid, and vitamin E.

132

Aluminium, stainless steel, glass and enamel are the best utensils for retaining nutrients while cooking. Iron pots can give you the benefit of that mineral, but they will shortchange you on vitamin C.

The shortest cooking time and the smallest amount of water are the least destructive to nutrients.

Milk in glass containers can lose riboflavin, as well as vitamins A and D, unless kept out of the light. Breads exposed to light can also lose these nutrients.

Well-browned, crusty, or toasted baked goods have less thiamine than others.

Bake and boil potatoes in their skins to get the most vitamins from them.

Use cooking water from vegetables to make soups, juices from meats for gravies, and syrups from canned fruits to make desserts.

Refrain from using any baking soda when cooking vegetables if you want to benefit from their thiamine and vitamin C.

Store vegetables and fruits in the refrigerator as soon as you bring them home from the market.

IX

Read the Label

The Importance of Understanding What's on Labels

All too often people buy supplements and never even look at the labels. They ask a clerk for a multivitamin and take what they are given, not realising that they might be getting short-changed on the vitamin content. All multivitamins differ in amounts included, and the most expensive tablet is not necessarily the best. The only way to be sure you're getting the B_6, folacin, or C that you need is to read the small print on the label. Also, if you have any allergies, it's wise to check what else you're getting with your supplement. [See Chapter IV.]

If there are words on the label that you don't understand, ask the pharmacist or assistant to explain them. If they can't, buy your supplements where someone can. And above all, remember to check the dosage you're getting. If you've been instructed to take vitamin E four times a day, it's unlikely that you want 400 IU. Vitamins and minerals come in different strengths. Be sure you're getting what you ask for — and need. Not understanding labels can often negate a lot of vitamin benefits.

How Does That Measure Up?

The terminology for measuring vitamin activity is not as confusing as you might think. Fat-soluble vitamins [A, E, D, and K] are usually measures in International Units [IU]. Recently, though, an expert committee of the Food and Agriculture Organisation/World Health Organisation [FAO/WHO] decided to change this order of measurement for vitamin A. Instead of using International Units, they proposed that vitamin A be evaluated in terms of retinol equivalents [RE], that is, the equivalent weight of retinol [vitamin A_1, alcohol] *actually absorbed and converted*.

Retinol equivalents come out to about five times less than International Units [IU]. Recommended allowances of 5,000 IU for a male between the ages of twenty-three and fifty would only be 1,000 RE; 4,000 IU for similarly aged females would only be 800 RE.

Most other vitamins and minerals are measured in milligrams [mg.] and micrograms [mcg.]. If you know that 1 g. equals .035 ounce, that it takes 28.35 g. to equal 1 ounce [and 1 fluid ounce equals 2 tablespoons], you'll have a better idea of just how much — or rather, how little — it takes for vitamins and minerals to do their job. The following table is a handy guide to refer to:

What's What in Weights and Measures

Metric Measure

1 kilogram equals 1,000 grams
1 gram equals 1,000 milligrams

1 milligram equals 1/1,000th part of a gram
1 microgram equals 1/1,000th part of a milligram
1 gamma equals 1 microgram

Avoirdupois Weight

16 ounces equal 1 pound
7,000 grains equal 1 pound
453.6 grams equal 1 pound
1 ounce av. equals 437.5 grains
1 ounce av. equals 28.35 grams

Conversion Factors

1 gram equals 15.4 grains
1 grain equals 0.065 grams [65 milligrams]
1 ounce apothecary equals 31.1 grams
1 fluid ounce equals 29.8 cc.
1 fluid ounce equals 480 minims

Liquid Measure

1 drop equals 1 minim
1 minim equals 0.06 cc.
15 minims equal 1.0 cc.
4 cc. equals 1 fluid dram
30 cc. equals 1 fluid ounce

Household Measure

1 teaspoon equals 4 cc. equals 1 fluid dram
1 tablespoon equals 15 cc. equals ½ fluid ounce
½ pint equals 240 cc. equals 8 fluid ounces

Abbreviations

AMDR	Adult Minimum Daily Requirement
USP Unit	United States Pharmacopoeia
BPC	British Pharmacopoeia
IU	International Unit
MDR	Minimum Daily Requirement
mg.	milligram
mcg.	microgram
g.	gram
gr.	grain

Breaking the RDA Code

Many people are bewildered by the variances between vitamin standards listed as RDA, U.S. RDA, and MDR. It becomes much less confusing when you understand that they are not the same thing.

RDA [*Recommended Daily Dietary Allowances*] came into being in 1941, when the Food and Nutrition Board of the National Research Council of the Academy of Sciences of the United States was established by the government to safeguard public health. The RDA are not formulated to cover the needs of those who are ill — they are not therapeutic and are meant strictly for healthy individuals — nor do they take into account nutrient losses that occur during processing and preparation. They are *estimates of* nutritional needs necessary to ensure satisfactory growth of children and the prevention of nutrient depletion in adults. *They are not meant to be optimum intakes, nor are they recommendations for an ideal diet.* They are not average requirements but recommendations intended to meet the needs of those *healthy* people with the highest requirements.

U.S. RDA [*U.S. Recommended Daily Allowances*] were formulated by the Food and Drug Administration [FDA] to be used as the legal standards for food labelling in regard to nutrient content. [The RDA were used as the basis for the U.S. RDA.] Calories and ten nutrients must be listed on food labels — protein, carbohydrate, fat, vitamin A, vitamin C, thiamin, riboflavin, niacin, calcium, and iron. Because the U.S. RDA are based on the highest values of the RDA, the former is frequently higher than the basic needs of most healthy people, though very few individuals today fall into that hypothetical category. Individuals vary by wide margins, and stress and illness, past and present, affect everyone differently. As far as I am concerned [and many other leading nutritionists], the RDA and U.S. RDA are *woefully inadequate*.

MDR [*Minimum Daily Requirements*] were the first set of standards established by the FDA and have been revised and replaced by the U.S. RDA.

What to Look For

As noted, when buying minerals, look for *chelated* on the label. Only 10 percent of ordinary minerals will be assimilated by the body, but when combined with amino acids in chelation, the assimilation is three to five times more efficient.

Hydrolysed means water dispersible. *Hydrolysed protein-chelate* means the supplement is in its most easily assimilated form.

Predigested protein is protein that has already been broken down and can go straight to the bloodstream.

Cold pressed is important to look for when buying oil or oil capsules. It means vitamins haven't been destroyed by heat, and that the oil, extracted by cold-pressed methods, remains polyunsaturated.

X

Fat and Fat Manipulators

Lipotropics — What Are They?

Methionine, choline, inositol and betaine are all lipotropics, which means their prime function is to prevent abnormal or excessive accumulations of fat in the liver.

Lipotropics also increase the liver's production of lecithin, which keeps cholesterol more soluble, detoxifies the liver, and increases resistance to disease by helping the thymus gland to carry out its functions.

Who Needs Them and Why

We all need lipotropics, some of us more than others. Anyone on a high-protein diet falls into the latter category. Methionine and choline are *necessary* to detoxify the amines that are by-products of protein metabilism.

Because nearly all of us consume too much fat [the average consumption in the United States is now 40 to 45 percent of total calories], and a good part of that is saturated fat, lipotropics are indispensable. By helping the liver produce lecithin, they're helping to keep cholesterol from forming dangerous deposits in blood vessels, lessening chances of heart attacks, arteriosclerosis, and gallstone formation as well.

Lipotropics keep cholesterol moving safely. We also need lipotropics to stay healthy, since they aid the thymus in stimulating the production of antibodies, the growth and action of phagocytes [which surround and gobble up invading viruses and microbes], and in destroying foreign or abnormal tissue.

Cholesterol

Like everything else, there's a good and bad side to fats. The general misconception that all of them are bad for you, prevalent as it may be, simply is not true. And the most maligned of all is cholesterol.

Practically everyone knows that cholesterol can be responsible for arteriosclerosis, heart attacks, a variety of illnesses, but very few are aware of the ways that it is *essential* to health.

At least two-thirds of your body cholesterol is produced by the liver or in the intestine. It is found there as well as in the brain, the adrenals, and nerve fibre sheaths. And when it's good, it's very, very good:

> Cholesterol in the skin is converted to essential vitamin D when touched by the sun's ultraviolet rays.
> Cholesterol aids in the metabolism of carbohydrates. [The more carbohydrates ingested, the more cholesterol produced.]
> Cholesterol is a prime supplier of life-essential adrenal steroid hormones, such as cortisone, and sex hormones.

New research shows that cholesterol behaves differently depending on the protein to which it is bound. Lipoproteins are the factors in our blood which transport cholesterol. Low-density lipoproteins [LDL] carry about 65 percent of blood cholesterol, very-low-density lipoproteins [VLDL] about 15 percent, and do seem to bear a correlation to heart disease. But high-density lipoproteins [HDL], which carry about 20 percent, appear to have the opposite effect. HDL are composed principally of lecithin, whose detergent action breaks up cholesterol and can transport it easily through the blood without clogging arteries. Essentially, the higher your HDL, the lower your chances of developing symptoms of heart disease.

It's interesting to note that females, who live eight years longer than males on the average, have higher HDL levels, and surprisingly, so do moderate alcohol drinkers.

Eggs might not be as bad as you thought. It is also worth mentioning for instance that though the egg consumption in the United States is one-half of what it was in 1945, there has *not* been a comparable decline in heart disease. And though the American Heart Association deems eggs hazardous, a diet without them can be equally hazardous. Not only do eggs have the most perfect protein components of any food, but they contain lecithin, which aids in fat assimilation. And, most important, they *raise* HDL levels!

How to Raise and Lower Cholesterol Levels

RAISE CHOLESTEROL	LOWER CHOLESTEROL
Cigarettes	Aubergine
Food additives such as BHT	Onions [raw or cooked]
Pollutants such as PCBs	Garlic
Coffee	Yoghurt [even made from whole
Stress	milk]
The pill	Pectin [unpeeled apple, scraped
Refined sugar	apple, white membrane of citrus
	fruits]
	soyabeans

For cholesterol watchers, a meal of light-meat turkey is a good choice, especially since no more than 300 mg. of cholesterol a day are recommended for the average person. Three ounces of light-meat turkey have only about 67 mg. cholesterol [though the same amount of dark meat has 75 mg.] Be careful of turkey liver, though; one cup of it, chopped, has about 839 mg. And remember, vegetables are cholesterol-free without butter.

XI

Carbohydrates and Enzymes

Why Carbohydrates Are Necessary

Carbohydrates, the scourge of misinformed dieters, are the main suppliers of our body's energy. During digestion, starches and sugars, the principal kinds of carbohydrates, are broken down into glucose, better known as blood sugar. This blood sugar provides the essential energy for our brain and central nervous system.

You need carbohydrates in your daily diet so that vital tissue-building protein is not wasted for energy when it might be needed for repair.

They have the same calories as protein. If you eat too many carbohydrates, more than can be converted into glucose or glycogen [which is stored in liver and muscles], the result, as we know all too well, is fat. When the body needs more fuel, the fat is converted back to glucose and you lose weight.

Don't be too down on carbohydrates. They're as important for good health as other nutrients — and gram for gram they have the same 4 calories as protein. Though no official requirement exists, a minimum of 50 g. daily is recommended to avoid ketosis, an acid condition of the blood that can happen when your own fat is used primarily for energy.

The Truth About Enzymes

Enzymes are necessary for the digestion of food, releasing valuable vitamins, minerals, and amino acids which keep us alive and healthy.

Enzymes are catalysts, meaning they have the power to cause an internal action without themselves being changed or destroyed in the process.

Enzymes are destroyed under certain heat conditions.

Enzymes are best obtained from uncooked or unprocessed fruits, vegetables, eggs, meats, and fish.

Each enzyme acts upon a specific food; one cannot substitute for the other. A deficiency, shortage, or even the absence of one single enzyme can mean the difference between sickness and health.

Enzymes that end in *-ase* are named by the food substance they act upon. For example, with phosphorus the enzyme is called phosphatase; with sugar [sucrose] it is known as sucrase.

Pepsin in a vital digestive enzyme that breaks up the proteins of ingested food, splitting them into usable amino acids. Without pepsin, protein could not be used to build healthy skin, strong skeletal structure, rich blood supply, and strong muscles.

Renin is a digestive enzyme which causes coagulation of milk, changing its protein, casein, into a usable form in the body. Renin releases the valuable minerals from milk, calcium, phosphorus, potassium, and iron that are used by the body to stabilise the water balance, strengthen the nervous system, and produce strong teeth and bones.

Lipase splits fat, which is then utilised to nourish the skin cells, protect the body against bruises and blows, and ward off the entrance of infectious virus cells and allergic conditions.

Hydrochloric acid in the stomach works on tough foods such as fibrous meats, vegetables, and poultry. It digests protein, calcium, and iron. Without HC1, problems such as pernicious anaemia, gastric carcinoma, congenital achlorhydria, and allergies can develop. Because stress, tension, anger, and anxiety before eating, as well as deficiencies of some vitamins [B complex primarily] and minerals, can all cause a lack of HC1, more of us are short of it than realise it. If you think you have an over-acid problem or heartburn, for which you are dosing yourself with an antacid such as Alka-Seltzer, you are probably unaware that *the symptoms of having too little acid are exactly the same as having too much*, in which case the taking of antacids, could be the worst possible thing for you to do.

Dr. Alan Nittler, author of *A New Breed of Doctor*, has stated emphatically that everyone over the age of forty should be using a HC1 supplement.

Betaine HCl and glutamic acid HCl are the best forms of commercially available hydrochloric acid.

The Twelve Tissue Salts and Their Functions

Tissue salts are inorganic mineral components of your body's tissues. They are also known as Schuessler biochemical cell salts, after Dr. W.H. Schuessler, who isolated them in the late nineteenth century. Dr. Schuessler found that if the body was deficient in any of these salts, illness occurred, and that if the deficiency was corrected, the body could heal itself. In other words, tissue salts are *not a cure*, but merely a remedy.

The twelve tissue salts are:

Fluoride of lime [calc. fluor.] — Part of all the connective tissues in your body. An imbalance can be the cause of varicose veins, late dentition, muscle tendon strain, carbuncles, and cracked skin.

Phosphate of lime [calc. phos.] —Found in all your body's cells and fluids, an important element in gastric juices as well as bones and teeth. An imbalance or deficiency can be the cause of cold hands and feet, numbness, hydrocele, sore breasts, and night sweats.

Sulphate of lime [calc. sulph.] — A constituent of all connective tissues in minute particles, as well as in the cells of the liver. An imbalance or deficiency can be the cause of skin eruptions, deep abscesses, or chronic oozing ulcers.

Phosphate of iron [ferr. phos.] — Part of your blood and other body cells, with the exception of nerves. An imbalance or deficiency can be the cause of continuous diarrhoea or, paradoxically, constipation. It has also been used as a remedy for nose-bleeds and excessive menses.

Chloride of potash [kali. mur.] — Found in lining and under the surface body cells. An imbalance or deficiency can be the cause of granulation of the eyelids, blistering eczema, and warts.

Sulphate of potash [kali. sulph.] — The cells that form your skin and internal organ linings interact with this salt. An imbalance or deficiency can be the cause of skin eruptions, a yellow coating on the back of the tongue, feelings of heaviness, and pains in the limbs.

Potassium phosphate [kali. phos.] — Found in all your body tissues, particularly nerve, brain, and blood cells. An imbalance or deficiency can be the cause of improper fat digestion, poor memory, anxiety, insomnia, and a faint, rapid pulse.

Phosphate of magnesia [mag. phos.] — Another mineral element of bones, teeth, brain, nerves, blood, and muscle cells. An imbalance or deficiency can be the cause of cramps, neuralgia, shooting pains, and colic.

Chloride of soda [nat. mur.] —Regulates the amount of moisture in the body and carries moisture to cells. An imbalance or deficiency can be the cause of salt cravings, hay fever, watery discharges from eyes and nose.

Phosphate of soda [nat. phos.] — Emulsifies fatty acids and keeps uric acid soluble in the blood. An imbalance or deficiency can be the cause of jaundice, sour breath, an acid or coppery taste in the mouth.

Sulphate of soda [nat. sulph.] — A slight irritant to tissues and functions as a stimulant for natural secretions. An imbalance or deficiency can be the cause of low fevers, edema, depression, and gallbladder disorders.

Silicic acid [silicea] — Part of all connective tissue cells, as well as those of the hair, nails, and skin. A deficiency or imbalance can be the cause of poor memory, carbuncles, falling hair, and ribbed, ingrowing nails. Eating whole-grain products should supply the normal need for this tissue salt.

PART TWO

GETTING YOURS

XII

Your Special Vitamin Needs

Selecting Your Regimen

We all know that not everyone has the same metabolism, but we often forget that this also means that not everyone requires the same vitamins. In the following sections I have outlined a number of personalised regimens for a variety of specialised needs. Look them all over and see which ones best fit your own special situation. If you fall under more than one category, adjust the combined regimens so that you are not double-dosing yourself, only adding the additional vitamins.

You will notice that in many cases I advise what I call an nsp, a nutrition starter programme. This basic vitamin trio, taken twice daily, is my foundation for general good health.

nsp nutrition starter programme

High-potency multiple vitamin with chelated minerals [time release preferred]

Vitamin C, 1,000 mg. with bioflavonoids, rutin, hesperidin, and rose hips.

High-potency chelated multiple minerals, 1 of each with breakfast and dinner.

Please note: Before starting any programme you should check "Cautions" [Chapter XXIII] and with a nutritionally orientated doctor – *the regimens in this book are not prescriptive nor are they intended as medical advice.*

Women

12–18 Multiple vitamin and mineral
      Vitamin C, 500 mg. with rose hips
      Vitamin E, 200 IU [dry form]
      1 of each with breakfast

19–50 High-potency multiple vitamin and mineral [time release preferred]
Vitamin C, 1,000 mg. with bioflavonoids
Vitamin E, 400 IU [dry form]
1 of each with breakfast, and again with evening meal if necessary
Also, 3 RNA–DNA, 100 mg. tablets daily
3 S.O.D. tablets daily (for 6 days a week only)
1 multiple digestive enzyme when needed
Stress B complex A.M. and P.M. if stress conditions exist

50+ Multiple vitamin and mineral [time release preferred]
Vitamin C, 1,000 mg. with bioflavonoids
Vitamin E, 400 IU [dry form]
1 of each with breakfast; repeat at evening meal if desired
3 RNA–DNA 100-mg. tablets daily
2 multiple minerals daily
1–3 multiple digestive enzymes daily

Men

11–18 Multiple vitamin and mineral
Vitamin C, 500 mg. with rose hips
Vitamin E, 400 IU [dry form]
1 of each with breakfast

19–50 High-potency multiple vitamin and mineral [time release preferred]
Vitamin C, 1,000 mg. with bioflavonoids
Vitamin E, 400 IU [dry form]
1 of each A.M. and P.M.
3 RNA–DNA 100-mg. tablets daily
3 S.O.D. tablets (daily for 6 days a week only)
2 multiple minerals
Lecithin granules, 2tbsp. or 9 capsules daily
Stress B complex A.M. and P.M. if needed

50+ Multiple vitamin and mineral
Vitamin C, 1,000 mg. with bioflavonoids
Vitamin E, 400 IU [dry form]

1 of each twice a day
3 RNA–DNA 100-mg. tablets daily
2 multiple minerals
1–3 multiple digestive enzymes daily

Infants

1–4   One good-tasting chewable multiple vitamin daily [check label to see that all the primary vitamins are included]; there should be no artificial colour, flavours, or sugar [sucrose] added.

Children

4–12   Growing children need a strong multiple vitamin containing minerals, especially calcium and iron, for normal growth. The tablet should also be high in B complex and vitamin C. One daily is sufficient [check label to be sure there is no artificial colour, flavour, or sugar [sucrose] added.

Pregnant Women

The right vitamins are essential at this time:

A good high-potency multiple vitamin and mineral rich in vitamins A, B_6, B_{12}, C, and folic acid.
Multiple chelated minerals, rich in calcium [2 tablets should equal 1,000 mg. calcium and 500 mg. magnesium]
1 of each twice daily
Also, folic acid, 800 mcg. 3 times a day

Nursing Mothers

The same supplements recommended for pregnant women plus additional vitamins A, B_6, B_{12}, and C. Your body and your baby need the best nourishment you can give them.

149

Runners

During the first fifteen to twenty minutes of running you burn up almost only glucose. The body then comes in with fats [lipids] for energy [in utilising lipids for energy, a compound called acetyl-coenzyme-A is formed]. If there are only animal fats present, the compound forms slowly and energy is insufficient. If polyunsaturates are present, on the other hand, the compound forms quickly. Increase your intake of polyunsaturates — seeds, peanuts – and antioxidants, such as vitamin A, C, E and selenium, to avoid free radical reactions.

A good supplement programme would be:

Multiple vitamin with chelated minerals
Vitamin C complex, 1,000 mg.
Stress B complex
1 of each 2–3 times a day
Also, vitamin E, 400 IU A.M. and P.M. and 1 multiple chealted mineral tablet daily.

Joggers

The nutritional needs of joggers are the same as those for runners. Just remember: for highest energy keep polyunsaturates in mind.

Executives

With tension and stress an accepted part of your daily life, and energy a necessity, you need a vitamin regimen that won't let you down. Many high-level executives I know use this one:

nsp A.B. and P.M.
Stress B complex A.M. and P.M.
Lecithin granules, 2 tbsp. or 3 capsules with each meal
B_{15}, 50 mg. 1–3 times daily.

If you're in a hurry in the morning, you might want to try my high-energy breakfast drink:

2 tbsp. protein powder
1tbsp. natural yeast
2tbsp. lecithin powder
3 ice cubes
2tbsp, fresh fruit, honey, or fructose

Mix in blender at high speed for one minute.

Students
Eating on the run, skipping breakfast, and not getting enough rest is a way of life for most students. And as if this isn't bad enough for good health, student diets usually consist of mostly starches and carbohydrates. If you're in this category, be aware that these factors, as well as your constant stress situations at school, are taking their toll. A good supplement programme would be:

nsp
Vitamin E, 400 IU
Stress B complex
1 of each with breakfast and dinner
Choline 100 mg 3 times daily

Also you might improve your work performance by increasing your intake of choline-rich foods.

Senior Citizens

The nutritional needs of senior citizens may vary widely, depending on the individual. As a general rule, however, if you're over sixty-five you need extra minerals, especially calcium, magnesium, and iron, as well as extra vitamins such as B complex and C. Vitamin E can help alleviate poor circulation, which is so often responsible for leg cramps. And don't forget about fibre. If chewing is a problem, high-fibre foods can be ground to convenient sizes or textures and are just as effective. Also, sweets should be discouraged, as their is a high incidence of sugar diabetes among older people.

151

A good supplement regimen would be:

Multiple vitamin and mineral
Rose hips vitamin C, 500 mg. with bioflavonoids
Multiple chelated mineral tablet
Vitamin E, 400 IU [dry form]
1 of each with breakfast and dinner

Athletes

Athletes have very demanding nutritional needs. The prime nutritional requirement for performance is energy, and high-energy foods — as opposed to "quick-energy" foods — should be eaten. If you're involved in action sports, you need a diet with more carbohydrates and protein than someone involved in a low-energy sport. Then again, even golf can become a high-energy game when carried on intensively for a long time. Keep in mind that excess amounts of glucose, sugar, honey or hard candy tend to draw fluid into the gastrointestinal tract. This can add to dehydration problems in endurance performance. A thirst-quenching tart drink of frozen or canned fruit juice is the best quick-energy beverage.

For supplements, I recommend:

Multiple vitamin and chelated minerals
Stress B complex
Vitamin C complex, 1,000 mg.
Vitamin E, 400-1,000 IU
Multiple chelated minerals
1 of each with breakfast, lunch, and dinner
Cytochrome-C and inosine
Vitamin B_{15}, 50 mg
Octacosanol 1–3 times daily

A protein supplement is also a good idea.

Night Workers

The Centre for Research on Stress and Health at the Stanford Research Institute has found that "the rotating shift exacts a heavy physical and emotional toll from workers." When eating and sleeping patterns are disrupted, so are the body's biological rhythms, and it takes "three to four weeks for the circadian rhythms to become synchronised." If you change from day to night shifts often, your body is under much stress, your chances of illness are greater, and your risk of ulcers is high. I feel that supplements are essential:

nsp
1 vitamin D, 400 IU with largest meal
3 tryptophan tablets half hour before bedtime [whenever that happens to be]

Lorry Drivers

Tension, stress, and a diet that is all too often high in greasy foods are important reasons for considering the following supplements.

nsp
1 B complex, 100 mg.
3 tryptophan tablets a half hour before bedtime if needed for sleep

Dancers

Dancers have energy requirements that rank with those of athletes, but because of weight restrictions they cannot consume the same amount of carbohydrates. Good supplements are indispensable, as most dancers will tell you. I suggest:

nsp [be sure to take the multiple mineral twice daily]
1 balanced calcium and magnesium supplement daily
B_{15}, 50 mg. 3 times daily

Building Workers

One out of every four workers is exposed to substances considered hazardous, according to the National Institute for Occupational Safety and Healthy [NIOSH]. Construction workers are particularly vulnerable. Depending upon the sort of construction you're doing and where you're doing it, you're exposed to a variety of harmful conditions from general pollution to inhaling lead oxide, which can happen if you're soldering scrap metal or plastics. In any event, a diet rich in antioxidants such as vitamins A, C, and E will help detoxify your body. The following supplements are recommended:

nsp
B complex, 100 mg. twice daily
Vitamin E, 400–1,000 IU twice daily

Salespeople

The daily grind of having to deal with the public cannot be underestimated. Whether you're selling automobiles, books, exercise machines, or food, doing it on the road or from behind a counter, the emotional and physical stress on your body is great. And because appearances are often as important as products in your line of work, your'd be wise to pack the right supplements along with your samples. You'll be happily surprised with the results.

nsp
Stress B complex 3 times daily [with each meal]
Vitamin E, 400 IU A.M. and P.M.

Actors

There's not an actor or actress I known who doesn't need a B-vitamin supplement. The stress and tension of performance is an occupational hazard. And if you're like most theatrical performers, dieting is the only form of eating you know, too often denying you necessary vitamins. The following supplements would be helpful:

nsp A.M and P.M.
Stress B complex A.M. and P.M.
Vitamin E, 400 IU twice daily

Singers

Like actors, singers are also under high levels of stress, whether performing or rehearsing. If you worry about laryngitis, or other throat infections, it's advisable to keep your vitamin-C levels high at all times. Time-release vitamin C is your best choice.

nsp
Additional vitamin C, 1,000 mg. A.M. and P.M. when necessary

Doctors and Nurses

If you work with illness, you need all the protection you can get. Long hours, stress, and germs themselves, all contribute to your need for vitamin and mineral supplementation.

nsp
Stress B complex twice daily
Extra vitamin C to ward off infections

Handicapped

If you are disabled, your needs for vitamins are usually increased. More often than not, if one part of your body is not functioning properly, another part is working twice as hard — and needs nourishment. Helpful basic supplements would be:

1 B complex, 50 mg. A.M. and P.M.
1 high-potency multiple mineral twice daily

Golfers

As much as you enjoy it, golfing takes a lot out of you. The stress and tension of the game can use up B vitamins at a rapid clip. The right supplements might not get you down into the seventies, but they can help you stay energetic throughout the game.

nsp
Stress B complex A.M. and P.M.

Tennis Players

If you play tennis often, you might look good on the outside, but be a nutritional mess inside. I've found that far too many tennis buffs skip meals, or eat only protein — both bad habits. A demanding game like tennis requires that you serve yourself all the vitamins you need.

nsp
Stress B complex A.M. and P.M.
Extra calcium to prevent muscle fatigue
Vitamin B_{15}, 50 mg. 1–3 times daily
Vitamin E, 400-1,000 IU daily
Wheat-germ oil
Liver-yeast supplement

Teachers

School days are as stressful for teachers as they are for students, if not more so. To keep your energy and spirits up, a good vitamin programme is important.

nsp A.M. and P.M.
Stress B complex twice daily

Smokers

Every cigarette you smoke destroys about 25 mg. of vitamin C. Also, lung cancer risk aside, you're more prone to cardiovascular and pulmonary disorders than nonsmokers. Without going into the long list of deleterious effects cigarettes can have, I feel confident in telling smokers that they need all the nutritional help they can get, especially from antioxidants such as vitamins A, C, E, and selenium.

nsp
Vitamin C, 2,000 mg. A.M. and P.M.
Vitamin E, 400–1,000 IU daily
Selenium, 50 mcg. 1–3 times daily
Vitamin A, 10,000 IU daily

Drinkers

Alcoholism is the chief cause of vitamin deficiency among civilised people with ample food supplies. If you're a heavy drinker, the alcohol you consume usually takes the place of needed protein, or, in some cases, prevents absorption or proper storage of ingested vitamins.

nsp
B complex, 100 mg. twice daily [especially needed are B_1, B_6, and folic acid]

Excessive TV Watchers

Just because you spend a lot of time relaxing in front of your seat doesn't mean you're not in need of extra vitamins. For the eyestrain it's more than likely that you need additional vitamin A. And if you rarely get to see the light of day, you might need vitamin D also.

nsp
Vitamin A, 10,000 IU with breakfast
Vitamin D, 400 IU 5 days a week if necessary

XIII

The Right Vitamin at the Right Time

Special Situation Supplements

Your body's vitamin needs are not always the same and special situations require special foods regimens and supplements. What follows is a list of such situations, most of them temporary, with supplement suggestions. For foods that offer specific vitamins and minerals see Chapters IV and V. Once again, this information is not prescriptive [See pages 119 for nsp.]

Acne

This scourge of teenage years has been treated in a variety of ways, from X-rays to tetracycline, with only varying degrees of success. I encourage more natural treatment of the condition, and have been delighted by the results.

Multiple vitamin *with* minerals but low in iodine, 1 daily
Vitamin E, 400 IU [dry form], 1–2 daily
Vitamin A, 25,000 IU [water soluble], 1–2 daily, 6 days a week
Zinc, 50 mg. chelated, 1 tablet 3 times daily with meals
Acidophilus liquid, 1–2 tbsp, 3 times daily, or 3–6 capsules 3 times daily
Eliminate all processed foods as they are usually high in iodized salt

Athlete's Foot

Vitamin C powder or crystals applied directly to the affected areas seems to help this fungus infection. Keep your feet dry, and out of shoes as much as possible, until the infection clears.

Bad Breath

Along with proper brushing and flossing, you might try:

nsp
1 chlorophyll tablet or capsule 1–3 times daily
3 acidophilus capsules 3 times daily, or 1–2 tbsp. flavoured acidophilus
Zinc, 50 mg. 1–3 times daily

Baldness or Falling Hair

There are no guarantees, but many people report a definite diminution of hair *loss* with this regimen:

Stress B complex twice daily
Choline and inositol, 1,000 mg. of each daily
Daily jojoba oil scalp massage and shampoo
A multiple-mineral formula with 1,000 mg. calcium and 500 mg. magnesium, 1 daily

Bee Stings

The best thing to do about bee stings is to try to avoid them. Vitamin B_1 [thiamine] has been shown to be a fairly good insect repellent. Taken three times, daily, 100 mg. B_1 creates a smell at the level of your skin that insects do not like. If you're too late with the B_1, and do get stung, 1,000 mg. vitamin C could help ease the allergic reactions.

Bleeding Gums

The most effective vitamin therapy for bleeding gums is 1,000 mg. vitamin C complex, with bioflavonoids, rutin, and hesperidin, taken three times a day.

Broken Bones

If you've ever broken a bone, you know how frustrating it is waiting for it to mend. That feeling can be alleviated, and bone healing accelerated, by increasing your calcium and vitamin-D intakes. Daily doses of 1,000 mg. calcium and 400 IU vitamin D are good, or bonemeal tablets with vitamin D, 5 to 10 daily, would be equally effective.

Bruises

Vitamin C complex, 1,000 mg. with bioflavonoids, rutin, and hesperidin, taken three times daily will help prevent capillary fragility, those black-and blue marks that occur when the tiny blood vessels beneath the skin rupture.

Burns

The most important thing to do with a burn is to put cold water on it immediately. To stimulate wound healing effectively 50 mg. zinc daily has been found useful and is worth trying. Vitamin C complex, 1,000 mg. with bioflavonoids, taken in the morning and evening is recommended to prevent infections. Vitamin E, 1,000 IU used orally and topically can help prevent scarring.

Cold Feet

If you're embarrassed by wearing socks to bed all the time, you could try a good multimineral supplement with iodine twice a day, along with kelp tablets. The cold feet could be due to the fact that your thyroid glands are not producing enough thyroxin. Niacin and Vitamin E can also help the circulation.

Cold Sores and Herpes Simplex

Few things are more annoying than cold sores. The best supplement remedy I've discovered is:

Vitamin C complex, 1,000 mg. with bioflavonoids A.M. and P.M.
Lactobacilus acidophilus, 3 capsules 3 times a day
Vitamin-E oil, 28,000 IU applied directly to affected area
Lystine 3 g. (300 mg) 3 times daily in divided doses between
    meals (with water — no protein)

Constipation

Everyone is bothered by constipation at some time or other. Usually this is due to a lack of bulk in the diet or because of certain medications, such as codeine. Harsh laxatives can rob the body of nutrients, as well as cause rebound constipation and laxative dependency, so natural remedies should be your first choice.

2 tbsp, unprocessed bran flakes daily
3–9 bran tablets daily
1 tbsp, acidophilus liquid 3 times daily

160

A vegetable laxative and stool softener for a short time if necessary

Cuts

Vitamin C complex, 1,000 mg. with bioflavonoids twice daily, along with 50 mg. zinc and 1,000 IU vitamin E.

Dry Skin

Vitamin-E oil seems to work wonders when applied to dry skin, as do oils rich in vitamin A and vitamin D. As a dietary supplement, if you're not eating enough sweet potatoes, carrots, liver, and tomatoes, try 25,000 IU vitamin A daily for two weeks, then cut dosage back to 10,000 IU. If you've cut all fats from your diet, put some back in the form of polyunsaturated oil. Two tablespoons on your daily salad is ample. Or try 3 to 6 lecithin capsules three times daily, along with nsp.

Hangovers

To prevent them, take 1 B complex, 100 mg. before going out, 1 again while you're drinking, and another right before going to bed. [Alcohol destroys B complex.]

If you already have one, take 1 B complex, 100 mg. three times daily. Portable oxygen works wonders.

Hay Fever

Stress can cause hay fever attacks to worsen. If you're one of the many who suffer, you might find relief with 1 stress B complex twice daily, pantothenic acid, 100 mg. three times daily, and extra vitamin C, which has evidenced effective antihistamine properties.

Headaches

A surprisingly effective vitamin-mineral regimen for headaches is:

100 mg. niacin 3 times daily
100 mg. stress B complex [time release] twice daily
Calcium and magnesium [twice as much calcium as magnesium is the proper ratio], which are nature's tranquillisers

Heartburn

Over-the-counter antacids contain aluminium, which disturbs calcium and phosphorus metabolism. You'll probably be better off taking 5 bonemeal tablets daily [with food], multiple digestive enzymes one to three times daily, and drinking fluids before or after meals, *not* during.

Haemorrhoids

Just about half the people over fifty are afflicted by haemorrhoids. Improper diet, lack of exercise, and straining at stool are all contributing factors. And coffee, chocolate, cola, and cocoa are accessories to the discomfort by promoting anal itching. If you're bothered by haemorrhoids, 1 tablespoon of unprocessed bran three times a day is helpful, along with 1,000 mg. vitamin C complex twice a day for healing membranes, and 3 acidophilus capsules three times a day [or 1 to 2 tablespoons of acidophilus liquid one to three times a day]. Vitamin E oil (28,000 I.U. per ounce) may be applied to affected area with a cotton swab.

Insomnia

Barbiturates are strong sedatives and hypnotics that are too often prescribed for insomnia. Aside from being habit-forming and dangerous if mixed with other drugs, these barbiturates can also cause low calcium levels.

Tryptophan, on the other hand, is a natural amino acid that is essential to our bodies, and helps induce sleep.

An effective anti insomnia programme:

3 tryptophan tablets (500–667 mg) a half hour before bedtime
1 chelated calcium and magnesium tablet 3 times daily and 3 tablets a half hour before bedtime
Vitamin B_6 100 mg and niacinamide 100 mg work together to

produce the brain chemical serotonin essential for restful REM sleep

Milk, as you know, is a fine natural source of calcium, and turkey is a good source of tryptophan. An open-face turkey sandwich and a glass of warm milk before bedtime could be the sleep remedy of your life.

Itching

As an antihistamine, 2 1,000-mg. vitamin-C tablets [time release] in the morning and in the evening, with food, might be helpful. I would also recommend a stress B complex with breakfast and dinner, 100 mg. pantothenic acid one to three times daily, and vitamin-E cream applied to afflicted area three times daily.

Jet Lag

So your plane from London lands at 9 A.M. and you're supposed to be at a meeting at 10 A.M. No problem, except for the fact that as far as your body is concerned, it's still only 4 A.M. and you should be asleep. Your best bet is to help your system catch up with your schedule by giving it the vitamins it needs.

Stress B complex [time release] A.M. and P.M. [start while on the plane].

nsp with food, two during flights of 5 or more hours
Vitamin E, 400 IU twice daily

If you're feeling run-down, as well as tired, to be sure to take additional vitamin C.

Leg Pains

Increase your calcium. Try 1 chelated calcium and magnesium tablet with breakfast and dinner, along with a chelated multiple mineral. Vitamin E has been reported quite helpful in cases of charley horse. The most common doses for it are 400 to 1,000 IU vitamin E (dry form) one to three times daily.

163

Menopause

Because of the risks that have recently been brought to light about oestrogen, many women have been seeking other ways to relieve the discomforts of menopause. A good number of menopausal women have found that 400 IU vitamin E one to three times a day does indeed alleviate hot flushes. If you're at that time of life, nsp and a 600-mg. stress B complex twice a day also seem to help. 500 mgs each of ginseng and damiana seem to help too.

Menstruation

Between the cramps and the bloating menstruation is for most women a monthly annoyance. But this annoyance can dwindle down to a mere distraction once the discomfort is alleviated.

Vitamin B_6, 150 mg. 3 times daily [most effective as a natural diuretic]
B complex, 100 mg. [time release] A.M. and P.M.
nsp
Evening Primrose Oil 500 mgs. 3 times daily

Motion Sickness

This is one condition where remedies are most effective if taken beforehand. Vitamins B_1 and B_6 are the nutrients of choice [in fact, many prenatal anti-nausea preparations contain vitamin B_6]. Taking 100 mg. B complex the night before you leave the morning of your trip has been found to be effective by many queasy travellers. Ginger root capsules taken 3 times daily work also.

Muscle Soreness

For that ache-all-over feeling after a workout, or just general muscle soreness, I've seen many people find relief with vitamin E, 400 to 1,000 IU taken one to three times daily. A chelated multiple mineral in the morning and at night also has helped.

164

The Pill

If you take oral contraceptives, not only are you more vulnerable than other women to blood clots, strokes, and heart attacks, but you're also more likely to be deficient in zinc, folic acid, vitamins, C, B_6 and B_{12} [which accounts for much nervousness and depression among pill takers].

Supplements are important:

nsp
Zinc, 50 mg. chelated, 1–3 tablets daily
Folic acid, 800 mcg. 1–3 times daily
B_{12}, 2,000 mg. [time release], A.M.
B_6, 50 mg. 1–3 times daily

Polyps

These small annoying growths should definitely be seen by a doctor, and in most instances surgical removal is necessary. But as far as supplements go, Dr. Jerome J. DeCosse, professor and chairman of surgery at the Medical College of Wisconsin, used 3,000 mg. vitamin C [time release] daily on patients with polyps, and had noteworthy success with the treatment.

Postoperative Healing

After surgery, your body needs all the nutritional support it can get.

Vitamin E, 400 IU [dry form] 3 times daily
2 vitamin C complex, 1,000 mg. with bioflavonoids, hesperidin, and rutin A.M. and P.M.
High-potency multiple vitamin with chelated minerals A.M. and P.M.
High-potency multiple chelated mineral tablet A.M. and P.M.
Vitamin A, 10,000–25,000 IU 3 times daily for 5 days [stop for 2 days to prevent build up]
Chelated zinc 15–50 mg. daily

Prickly Heat

Much like itching, prickly heat seems to respond to the antihistamine properties of vitamin C.

Prostate Problems

Chronic prostitis, where inflammation of the gland is the case as opposed to infection, has been found to respond to treatment with zinc. [The prostate gland normally contains about ten times more zinc than any other organ in the body.] In many cases, symptoms have completely disappeared.

nsp
Zinc, 50 mg. 3 times daily
Vitamin F or lecithin capsules [1,200 mg.], 3 caps 3 times daily

Psoriasis

Though many jokes have been made about this disease, it is no laughing matter to the millions who suffer from it. No one treatment has been found to be totally effective, but the following has met with much success:

nsp
Vitamin A [water soluble], 10,000 IU 3 times daily for 6 days a
    week
B complex, 100 mg. [time released] A.M. and P.M.
Rose hips vitamin C, 1,000 mg. A.M. and P.M. [this is in addition
    to the vitamin C called for in the nsp]
Vitamin E [dry form], 400 IU 3 times daily
3 vitamin-F for licithin capsules 3 times daily
Increase protein [preferably animal source]

Stopping Smoking

It's no mean feat to stop smoking, and your body knows it. Those withdrawal symptoms are real. For the irritability that occurs, 1 tryptophan [667 mg.] tablet three times a day between meals seems to help. Also 1 B complex, 100 mg. [time release], taken with the evening meal and cysteine 100 mg daily. Don't forget the nsp.

Sunburn

A good sunscreening preparation should always be used before exposing yourself to the sun's untraviolet rays for any length of time. What most people don't realise is that the sun actually burns the skin, and bad burns can break the skin and leave it vulnerable to infection.

If it's too later for preventives, try this:

Aloe vera gel applied 3–4 times daily
A PABA cream or vitamin-E cream [20,000 IU] also applied 3–4 times daily
nsp
Additional vitamin C, 1,000 mg. A.M. and P.M. until burn heals

Teeth Grinding

People are usually unaware of grinding their teeth. It occurs more often in children than adults, and most often during sleep. NSP; B complex, 100 mg. A.M. and P.M.; and a few bonemeal tablets nightly before sleep can help.

Varicose Veins

Age, lack of exercise, and chronic constipation are contributing factors to varicose veins. Watching your diet and exercising regularly can do a lot toward preventing them. NSP with an extra 1,000 mg. vitamin C complex twice daily has been found to help, along with 400 to 800 IU vitamin E.

Vasectomy

Men with vasectomies are more susceptible to infections and would be wise to take an additional 1,000 mg. vitamin C complex daily, along with regular nsp diet supplementation. Extra zinc 15–50 mg. every day is also a good idea.

Warts

They don't come from handling frogs, but they do seem to disappear effectively when treated with vitamin-E oil. The most successful regimen appears to be 28,000 IU vitamin E applied externally one to two times daily and 400 IU vitamin E [dry form] taken internally three times a day. Vitamin C 1,000 mg. can help build up the body's immunity and possibly prevent warts altogether.

Any Questions About Chapter XIII?

You talk about digestive enzymes being helpful for heartburn. What are they and what do they do?

Enzymes, which can be purchased as supplements, can help your own digestive system assimilate the foods you eat. *Bromelain*, for instance, is a digestive enzyme from pineapple. *Cellulase* is an aid to digesting vegetable matter and breaking down food fibre. *Hydrochloric acid (HC1)* works in the stomach on tough foods, such as fibrous meats, vegetables, and poultry. (Betaine HC1 is the best form available.) *Lipase* assists in fat digestion and *mylase* dissolves thousands of times its own weight in starches so you can more easily assimilate them. *Papain* is a protein-digesting enzyme (from papaya), and *prolase* is a concentrated protein-digesting enzyme derived from papain.

Is there a specific reason for your recommending ginseng in the treatment of menopause?

Definitely. Since oestrogen replacement began in the 1960s, it has been linked to a 35% increase in uterine cancer. Ginseng contains estriol, an anticarcinogenic (cancer-fighting) variant of oestrogen.

XIV

Getting Well and Staying That Way

Why You Need Supplements During Illness

During illness the body is under stress. Cells are destroyed, exhausted adrenal glands deprived of nutrients are unable to function properly, and the body's stress-fighting team of vitamin C, B_6, folic acid, and pantothenic acid is severely depleted.

Because we require these vitamins to utilise effectively other nutrients and to keep our metabolism functioning all the time, our need for them is obviously increased when we're ill. And since we know that fever and stress rob our body of its most essential nutrients, the importance of supplements is self-evident.

Again, the following regimens are not intended as medical advice, only as a guide in working with your doctor.

Allergies

Allergies come in all shapes and sizes, with all sorts of symptoms, and you can contact them for just about anything. Nonetheless, they take their nutritional toll and supplements can help.

1 stress B complex with vitamin C 3 times daily
Pantothenic acid, 100 mg. 3 times daily
nsp

If you have an allergy, it would be a good idea to take a hard look at your present diet. Many allergies are caused by MSG, food colouring additives and preservatives.

Arthritis

Thousands upon thousands of people suffer from this painful chronic condition. Because it puts so much stress on the body, vitamin-mineral supplementation is really essential.

nsp
Extra vitamin C, 1,000 mg. 1–3 times a day [if you take a lot of
   aspirin, you're losing vitamin C]
B complex, 100 mg. 1–3 times a day
B_{12} up to 2,000 mcg. daily
Niacin up to 1 g. daily
1–3 yucca tabs 3 times daily
Pantothenic acid, 100 mg. 3 times daily
Vitamin A, 10,000 IU, and vitamin D, 400 IU, 1–3 capsules 3
   times daily [take for 5 days and stop for 2]
   or
Cod liver oil, 1–2 tbsp. 3 times daily [if capsules, 3 caps 3 times
   daily]. Again, take for 5 days and stop for 2

Asthma

Asthma is a chronic allergic condition that affects the bronchial
tubes. When an attack occurs, the muscle tissue of the tubes
constricts spasmodically, squeezing the air passages and causing
laboured breathing and a feeling of suffocation. Allergies,
heredity, and emotional stress have all been implicated as contributing factors to asthmatic conditions, but many nutrients have
been found to provide remarkable natural relief.

nsp A.M. and P.M.
Extra vitamin C, 1,000 mg. 1–3 times daily

(*Caution*: Vitamin C that is buffered with calcium ascorbate can
interfere with the action of tetracylines. A sodium ascorbate
form of vitamin C can be used with tetracyclines, but not if you
are on a sodium-restricted diet or taking steroids.)

Evening Primrose Oil, 2 500 mg. tablets, 3 times daily for 3 to 4
   months; then 1 tablet 3 times daily
   (If you are taking steroids, you won't benefit from EPO,
   because steroids interfere with EPO's action.)
Vitamin B_{15}, 50 mg., 1 tablet daily for one month, then twice
   daily for the second month, and 3 times daily in the third
   month.

170

(Severe cases may require two 50 mg. tablets 3 times daily with food. Decrease dosage when positive reaction occurs.)
Glandulars (adrenal gland concentrates) 1–3 times daily, but not at night, because they might cause insomnia.

(*Caution:* Glandulars should not be taken by anyone who is allergic to beef or pork.)

Vitamin A (water soluble) 10,000–25,000 IU daily
Vitamin B_2 (riboflavin) 100 mg., 3–4 times daily
Vitamin B_5 (pantothenic acid) 1,000–2,000 mg. daily
Vitamin B_6 (pyridoxine) 100–200 mg. 1–4 times daily
Vitamin E (dry form) 400–1,200 IU daily

Blood Pressure — High and Low

HIGH

The importance of keeping your blood pressure down cannot be overestimated, and there are a number of natural ways that can help.

Talk slower (fast talkers often don't breath properly and this can result in elevated blood pressure)
Reduce, if you are overweight (controlled, sensible dieting can significantly lower blood pressure in overweight individuals)
Decrease sodium and increase potassium in your diet
Decrease your sugar intake
Eliminate caffeine
Eat more onions and garlic
Stop smoking
Avoid stress or anxiety-provoking situations (jangling everyday noises, even loud televisions, can cause stress and elevate blood pressure.
Regular exercise (such as brisk walking) and adequate rest

Regimen

Lecithin granules, 3 tbsp. daily, or 3 caps 3 times daily
Potassium may be necessary if you are taking an antihyperten-

sive, but check with your doctor to be sure it's not contraindicated for your particular medication.

nsp

Calcium 1,000–1,500 mg. daily

Vitamin E, 100 IU daily and work up to higher strengths (check with your doctor)

Garlic perles (deodorized) 1–3 daily

Low

Low blood pressure, unless extreme, is a far better condition to have than its alternative. Nonetheless, hypotensives often suffer from dizziness and occasional fainting spells and blackouts.

Regimen

1–3 kelp tablets daily

(If you're taking thyroid medication, check with your doctor, as kelp might decrease the need for the amount you're currently taking.)

nsp

Bronchitis

This inflammation of the bronchial tube lining is quite common and extremely enervating. The stress it puts on the body is high, and even antibiotics are the bad guys as far as nutrients are concerned.

Vitamin A, 25,000 IU 1–3 times daily [take for 5 days then stop for 2]

Rose hips vitamin C, 1,000 mg. A.M. and P.M.

nsp

Vitamin E, 400 IU [dry form] 1–3 times daily

Water, 6–8 glasses daily

3 acidophilus caps 3 times daily or 1–2 tbsp. liquid 3 times daily

Chicken Pox

This childhood staple is caused by a virus closely related to that of

172

shingles. The fever and itching deplete a good amount of nutrients. Many mothers have found their children up and about
faster by adding the following supplements to their diets.

Rose hips vitamin C, 500 mg. 3 times daily
Vitamin E, 100–299 IU 1–3 times daily
Vitamin A, 10,000 Iu daily [check paediatrician for proper
   dosage according to age and weight]. Take for 5 days and stop
   for 2
Multivitamin and mineral A.M. and P.M.

Colds

No one pays too much attention to a cold, except the body which
pays plenty.

nsp
Rose hips vitamin C, 1,000 mg. 3 times daily
Vitamin A, 25,000 IU 1–3 times daily [take for 5 days and stop for
   2]
Vitamin E, 400 IU [dry form] 1–3 times daily
Water, 6–8 glasses daily
3 acidophilus capsules 3 times daily or 1–2 tbsp, liquid 3 times
   daily

Colitis

As a rule this illness is more common in women than men and
often triggered by emotional upset. Alternating diarrhoea and
constipation, as well as abdominal pain, are its distressing hall-
marks. Diet is of prime importance and vitamins are recommended.

nsp
Potassium, 99 mg. [elemental] 1–3 times daily
Sugarless cabbage juice [vitamin U], 1 glass 3 times daily
Water, 6–8 glasses daily
Aloe vera gel [for internal use], 1 tbsp. 3 times daily or 1–3
   capsules 3 times daily
3–6 acidophilus caps 3 times daily or 2 tbsp. liquid 3 times daily
1 tbsp. bran flakes 3 times daily or 3–6 bran tablets

Diabetes

What happens in diabetes, primarily, is that the pancreas fails to produce adequate insulin and the blood sugar rises uncontrollably. In mild cases diet alone can control the condition. [Beware of hidden sugars. In severe cases, replacement insulin is necessary. In all cases, the care of a physician is essential.

Supplements that have aided diabetics are:

nsp
Chromium, 1–2 mg. daily for 6 months
Glucose Tolerance Factor (GTF)
Chromium 50 mg. 3 times daily
Potassium, 99 mg. 3 times daily
Chelated zinc, 50 mg. 1–3 times daily
Water, 6–8 glasses daily

Eye Problems

From simple inflammations to refraction difficulties to serious diseases, eye problems should never be ignored, nor should visits to the ophthalmologist or optician be postponed. There are, however, generally beneficial supplements you can take.

Vitamin A, 10,000 IU 1–3 times daily [take for 5 days, then stop for 2]
B complex, 100 mg. [time release] A.M. and P.M.
Rose hips vitamin C complex, 500 mg. A.M. and P.M.
Vitamin E, 400 IU [dry form] A.M. and P.M.

Heart Conditions

With any heart condition, you should be under a doctor's care. Though the following supplements have been found to be quite safe and helpful, you should check with your physician to make sure they are not contraindicated in your particular case. (Vitamin E can increase the imbalance between the two sides of the heart for some people with rheumatic hearts.)

Vitamin B, 100 mg. (time release) A.M. and P.M.
Extra niacin, 100 mg. 1–3 times daily

Vitamin E (dry form) 400 IU, 1 daily
nsp
3 lecithin capsules or 3 tbsp, granules 3 times daily
Chrondroitin Sulphate A (CSA)
EPA and DHA

HEART ATTACK PREVENTION TACTICS

Decrease sugar and salt consumption.

Stop smoking.

Exercise regularly.

Watch your weight.

Practice relaxation techniques such as meditation and biofeedback to reduce stress.

Decrease intake of saturated fats, hydrogenated oils and cholesterol.

Eat more garlic, fresh fruit, and fish.

Increase your soy protein intake (use in place of animal protein whenever possible).

Get enough calcium and magnesium in your diet (supplements of 1,000 mg. calcium and 500 mg. magnesium daily are recommended).

Be sure you're getting enough vitamins C, B_6, and E.

Supplement lecithin in your diet.

Laughter is great medicine (not only does it release pent-up emotions and stress . . . it's fun and feels good, too).

Hypoglycaemia

Though many millions of people have it, this disease is one of the most undiagnosed. It is a condition of low blood sugar, and, like diabetes, presents a situation where the body is unable to metabolise carbohydrates normally. Since a hypoglycaemic's system overreacts to sugar, producing too much insulin, the key to raising blood sugar levels is not by eating rapidly metabolised carbohydrates but by eating more protein.

Recommended supplements:

Vitamin A and D capsules [10,000 and 400 IU 1–3 times daily for

5 days, then stop for 2
Vitamin C, 500 mg. with or after each meal
Vitamin E, 100–200 IU 3 times daily
B complex, 50 mg. 3 times daily
Vitamin F 1 capsule 3 times daily
Multiple mineral tab A.M. and P.M. [Niacin as needed and toler-
    ated.]
Pantothenic acid, 200 mg. 3 times daily
2 lecithin capsules [9 grains = 1,200 mg.] 3 times daily
Digestive enzymes if necessary
1 kelp tablet 3 times daily
3 acidophilus capsules or 1–2 tbsp. liquid 3 times daily
GTF chromium, 50 mg. 3 times daily

Impetigo

Caused by germs similar to those that cause boils — staphylococ-
cus or streptococcus — it occurs more in children than adults, but
no one is immune. It often results from scratching and infecting
insect bites, allowing the germs to get into broken skin.

Vitamin A and D capsules [10,000 and 400 IU] 1–3 times daily
    [reduce dose for child] for 5 days, then stop for 2
Vitamin E, 100–400 IU [dry form] once a day
Rose hips vitamin C, 500 mg. A.M. and P.M.

Measles

You can get measles at any age, though it's more common among
children. It is the most contagious of the communicable diseases.
There is now a preventive vaccine for it, but the virus still
manages to get a large number of the unprotected each year. The
disease and rash can be mild, or severe with a heavy cough. Your
body needs vitamins to help fight and recover from it.

Vitamin A, 10,000 IU [reduce dose for child] 1–3 times daily for 5
    days, then stop for 2
Rose hips vitamin C, 500–1,000 mg. A.M. and P.M.
Vitamin E, 200–400 IU [dry form] A.M. *or* P.M.

176

Mononucleosis

Commonly contracted by adolescents and young adults, mono [glandular fever] or "the kissing disease" as it is often called, can happen to anyone and can deplete the body of massive amounts of nutrients.

Diet is important and supplements are generally considered essential during the long convalescence.

nsp
Extra vitamin C, 1,000 mg. A.M. and P.M. for 3 months
Potassium, 99 mg. 3 times daily
B complex, 100 mg. [time release] A.M. and P.M.

Mumps

A vaccine for mumps exists, but the disease is still quite common and just as nutritionally debilitating. The virus can spread through the patient's entire system, involving not only the salivary glands but the testicles or ovaries, the pancreas, the nervous system, and sometimes even the heart.

Vitamin A, 10,000 IU [reduce dose for children] 1–3 times daily for 5 days, then stop for 2
Rose Hips vitamin C, 500–1,000 mg. twice daily
Vitamin E, 200–400 IU [dry form] daily

P.M.S. (Premenstrual Syndrome)

For two to ten days before the onset of menstruation, millions of women are affected by a wide range of physical discomforts and mood disorders — from bloating, depression, and insomnia to severe pains, uncontrolled rages, crying spells, and even suicidal depression. This is known as P.M.S., premenstrual syndrome.

FOODS AND BEVERAGES TO AVOID

Salt and salty foods
Licorice (it stimulates the production of aldosterone which causes further retention of sodium and water)
Cold foods and beverages (these adversely affect abdominal circulation and worsen cramping)

177

Caffeine in all forms
Caffeine increases the craving for sugar, wastes B vitamins, washes out potassium and zinc, and increases hydrochloric acid (HC1) secretions which can cause abdominal irritation.

Astringent dark teas (tannin binds important minerals and prevents absorption in the digestive tract)

Alcohol (adversely affects blood sugar, depletes magnesium levels, and can interfere with proper liver function, which can aggravate P.M.S.)

Spinach, beet greens, and other oxalate-containing vegetables (oxalates make minerals nonassimilable, difficult to be properly absorbed)

FOODS AND BEVERAGES TO INCREASE

Strawberries, watermelon (eat seeds), artichokes, asparagus, parsley and watercress (these are natural diuretics)

Raw sunflower seeds, dates, figs, peaches, bananas, potatoes, peanuts, and tomatoes (rich in potassium)

Try Dong Quai, it's an herb known as the female ginseng and can improve circulation, regulate liver function, and help remove excess water from the system.

Suggested supplements

Vitamin B_6, 50–300 mg. daily (work up from 50 mg. gradually) nsp

Magnesium, 500 mg. and calcium 250 mg. daily
   (Yes, with P.M.S. it is twice as much magnesium as calcium, because a magnesium deficiency causes many of the P.M.S. symptoms.)

Vitamin E (dry form), 100–400 IU daily

Pantothenic acid (vitamin B_5), 1,000 mg. (1 g.) daily

Evening Primrose Oil, 500 mg., 1–3 times daily

And exercise! Aside from the fact that this will improve abdominal circulation, perspiration helps remove excess fluids. Brisk walking for 30 minutes twice daily and/or swimming are highly recommended.

Shingles

Shingles [herpes zoster] is caused by a virus much like the one that causes chicken pox. But where chicken pox causes a general skin eruption, shingles usually erupts along a nerve path. Differences aside, the nutritional deficit caused by both diseases is high.

Vitamin A, 10,000–25,000 IU 1–3 times daily for 5 days, then stop for 2
Vitamin B complex, 100 mg. [time release] A.M. and P.M.
Rose hips vitamin C with bioflavonoids, 1,000–2,000 mg. A.M. and P.M.
Vitamin D, 1,000 IU 1–3 times daily for 5 days, then stop for 2

Tonsillitis

An inflammation of the tonsils that can afflict any age group, though it is more common in children. Good nutrition and supplements have been effective in preventing it as well as recovering from it.

nsp
Vitamin A, 10,000–25,000 IU [reduce dose for children] 1–3 times daily for 5 days, then stop for 2
Extra vitamin C complex, 1,000 mg. A.M. and P.M.
Vitamin E, 400 IU [dry form] 1–3 times daily
3 acidophilus caps or 1–2 tbsp, 3 times daily
Water, 6–8 glasses daily

Ulcers

There are two types of peptic ulcer, one in the stomach and the other in the duodenum, usually associated with excessive acidity in the stomach juices. For both of these conditions, supplements have been found helpful.

Vitamin A, 25,000 IU 1–3 times daily for 5 days, then stop for 2
Vitamin B complex, 100 mg. [time release] A.M. and P.M.
Rose hips vitamin C with bioflavonoids, 1,000 mg. [time release] A.M. and P.M.

179

High-potency multiple mineral A.M. and P.M.
Aloe vera gel, 1–3 capsules or 1–3 tbsp. liquid daily

Venereal Disease

Syphilis and gonorrhoea are the main types of venereal disease. Sulphur drugs, penicillin, tetracycline, erythromycin, and the newer antibiotics, are the most effective treatments for them, but these remedies cause almost as much need for supplements as the diseases themselves.

nsp
3 acidophilus capsules or 1–2 tbsp. liquid 3 times daily
Extra rose hips vitamin C, 1,000 mg. A.M. and P.M.
Vitamin K, 100 mcg. daily if on extended antibiotic programme

Genital herpes has become the most widespread venereal disease of the '80s. Like herpes simplex type I, which causes cold sores, type II herpes, which causes genital infection, also seems to respond well to lysine-rich foods. As a preventative, it wouldn't be a bad idea to increase your intake of cottage cheese, flounder, tuna fish, peanuts, raw chick peas (garbanzos), and soybeans. *Acyclovir* is a drug that — at this writing — seems to be effective in blocking herpes replication, but the final results are not yet established for certain. Meanwhile, I'd suggest a preventative supplement of lysine, 500 mg. daily (with water or juice — no protein) and vitamin C, 1,000 mg. A.M. and P.M. If you already have the virus: lysine, 3 g. (3,000 mg.) 3 times daily – in divided doses — between meals.

IMPORTANT: If you have symptoms of herpes simplex virus I or II, avoid supplementation of arginine and argine-rich foods.

XV

It's Not All in Your Mind

How Vitamins and Minerals Affect Your Moods

The first scientifically documented discovery to relate mental illness to diet occurred when it was found that pellagra [with its depression, diarrhoea, and dementia] could be cured with niacin. After that, it was shown that supplementation with the whole B complex produced greater benefits than niacin alone.

Evidence of biochemical causes for mental disturbances continues to mount. Experiments have shown that symptoms of mental illness can be switched off and on by altering vitamin levels in the body.

Dr. R. Shulman, reporting in the *British Journal of Psychiatry*, found that forty-eight out of fifty-nine psychiatric patients had folic-acid deficiencies. Other research has shown that the majority of the mentally and emotionally ill are deficient in one or more of the B-complex vitamins or vitamin C. And even normal, happy people have been found to become depressed and experience other symptoms of emotional disturbance when made niacin or folic-acid deficient.

At California's Stanford University, Nobel Laureate Dr. Linus Pauling conducted a series of tests to determine individual vitamin needs. As part of the series, he administered massive doses of vitamin C [as much as 40 g.] to schizophrenics and discovered that little or none of it was discarded in the urine. Since the body expels what is doesn't need of the water-soluble vitamins, the test clearly indicated that the mentally ill needed more vitamin C — more than one thousand times the RDA — than the rest of us.

Vitamins and Minerals for Depression and Anxiety

The following vitamins and minerals have in many cases been

181

found to be effective in the treatment of depression and anxiety.

Vitamin B_1 [thiamine] — large amounts appear to energise depressed people and tranquilise anxious ones

Vitamin B_6 [pyridoxine] — important for the function of the adrenal cortex

Pantothenic acid — has a tension-relieving effect.

Vitamin C [Ascorbic acid] — essential for combatting stress

Vitamin E [alpha-tocopherol] — aids brain cells in getting their needed oxygen

Zinc — oversees body processes and aids in brain function

Magnesium — necessary for nerve functioning, known as the antistress mineral

Calcium — makes you less jumpy, more relaxed.

Other Drugs Can Add to Your Problems

Alcohol is a nerve depressant. If you take tranquillisers and a drink, the combination of the two can cause a severe depression — or even death.

If you take Darvon with a tranquilliser, you might find yourself experiencing tremors and mental confusion. The same thing can happen if you combine a sedative with an antihistamine [such as any found in over-the-counter cold preparations].

Oral contraceptives deplete the body of B_6, B_{12}, folic acid, and vitamin C. If you're on the pill and depressed, it is not surprising. Your need for B_2, necessary for normal tryptophan metabolism, is fifty to a hundred times a non-pill-user's requirement.

Drugs that you Might Not Think Would Cause Depression — But Can:

adrenocorticoids
baclofen
beta-blockers
antihypertensives
oestrogens
anti-arthritis medicines
potassium supplements
procainamide

propoxphene
any sex hormones
trimethobenzamide

XVI

Environmental Pollution and You

The Worst Things in Life Are Free

You still have some control over the food you eat and the water you drink, but you're stuck with the air you breathe. And if you live in any major urban area today, you're breathing polluted air.

With each breath you subject your lungs and body to a wide range of pollutants. No part of you is immune. Pollutants affect your nose, eyes, throat, skin, and internal organs as well. In fact, it has been estimated that breathing air in the Los Angeles basin is equivalent to smoking a pack of cigarettes a day. And since each cigarette is estimated to cut twelve minutes off your life, every breath you take in a polluted environment brings you that much closer to where you don't want to go.

Every year 200 million tons of potentially dangerous pollutants are released into the atmosphere. From industrial processes, incinerators, automobiles, fossil-fuel burning operations, electric power plants, refineries, and more, we are inundated with dust, smoke, fumes, gasses, and tiny particles of solid matter such as tars and poisonous heavy metals. And in one breath you can take in 70,000 such solid particles!

How does your body hold up against this kind of assault. Well, vitamins are your first line of defence. Especially the antioxidants — vitamins A, C, E, and selenium. These nutrients are capable of protecting other substances from oxidation. In other words, the free radicals [uncontrolled oxidations that damage cells] that are formed when we inhale pollutants are kept in check.

Know Your Antioxidants

Vitamin A protects mucous membranes of mouth, nose, throat, and lungs. It also helps protect vitamin C from oxidation, which allows your C to work better.

Vitamin C fights bacterial infections and reduces the effects of allergy-producing substances. It also protects vitamins A, E, and some of the B complex from oxidation.

Vitamin E protects vitamins B and C from oxidation. It has the ability to unite with oxygen and prevent it from being converted into toxic peroxides. It acts as an antipollutant for the lungs.

Selenium and vitamin E must both be present to corrext a deficiency in either. The levels of selenium in the blood of people in various cities has been found to bear a direct relationship to cancer mortality. The higher the levels of selenium, the lower the cancer death rate — and vice versa.

On-the-Job Dangers

The following is a list of work-related risks you might now know that you're taking:

Electrical engineers, electricians, and printers Exposure to electronic devices, fluorescent lights, disinfectants, measuring devices, or certain dyes and inks may subject you to an odourless mercury that can cause emotional disorders or even death.

Secretaries and receptionists Certain duplicating machines give off fumes that may cause visual problems, fatigue, and headaches. Some switchboards can release ozone, a colourless vapour that may cause respiratory disorders.

Paperhangers There are wallpapers coated with vinyl chloride, apparently carcinogenic, a chemical that can easily be inhaled.

Dentists, dental hygienists The silver amalgam, often used for fillings, contains mercury and can give off vapours. The Institute for Occupational Safety estimates that there are unheal-

184

thy levels of mercury in one out of every ten dentists' offices.

Mechanics   If you work with machinery that is cleaned by solvents, you can inhale vapours that may be injurious to your health, causing skin inflammations as well as liver and kidney disturbances.

Asbestos workers   It is estimated that 45 percent of asbestos-insulation workers will die of some form of cancer. [Breathing in buildings where asbestos has been sprayed on steel beams and may flake off could be dangerous to anyone's health.]

Workers in any of these occupations should be taking supplemental antioxidants daily: Vitamins A, C, E and Selenium.

Have you taken an antioxidant today?

PART THREE

VITAMINS VS. DRUGS

XVII

Drugs and You

Effects of Caffeine on the Body

There are no doubts about it, caffeine is a powerful drug. That's right, *drug*. Chances are you're not just enjoying your daily coffees or colas, you're addicted to them.

Caffeine acts directly upon the central nervous system. It brings about an almost immediate sense of clearer thought and lessens fatigue. It also stimulates the release of stored sugar from the liver, which accounts for the "lift" coffee, cola, and chocolate [the caffeine big three] give. But these benefits may be far outweighed by the side effects.

The release of stored sugar places heavy stress on the endocrine system.

Heavy coffee drinkers often develop nervousness or become jittery.

Coffee-drinking housewives demonstrated symptoms typical of drug withdrawal when switched to a decaffeinated beverage.

Dr John Minton, professor of surgery at Ohio State University and specialist in cancer oncology, has found that excessive intake of methylxanthines [active chemicals in caffeine] can cause benign breast disease and prostate problems.

Many doctors consider caffeine a culprit in hypertensive heart disease.

Dr Phillip Cole, in the British medical journal *The Lancet*, reported a strong relationship between coffee consumption and cancer of the bladder and the lower urinary tract.

People who drink five cups of coffee daily have a 50 percent greater chance of having heart attacks than non-coffee drinkers, according to the *British Medical Journal*.

The *Journal of the American Medical Association* reports a

disease called caffeinism, with symptoms of appetite loss, weight loss, irritability, insomnia, feelings of flushing chills, and some times a lower fever.

Scientists at John Hopkins University have shown that caffeine can interfere with DNA replication.

The Centre for Science in the Public Interest advises pregnant women to stay away from caffeine, since studies have shown that the amount contained in about four cups of coffee per day causes birth defects in test animals.

High doses of caffeine will cause laboratory animals to go into convulsions and then die.

Caffeine can be highly toxic [the lethal dose estimated to be around 10 g.]. New research shows that the one quart of coffee consumed in three hours can destroy much of the body's thiamine.

You're Getting More Than You Think

The following table shows the amount of caffeine [in milligrams] consumed in specific beverages and drugs:

BEVERAGE	12-OUNCE CAN or BOTTLE
Pepsi-Cola	43.1 mg.
Coca-Cola	64.7 mg.
Coffee	*Per Serving*
Instant	66.0 mg.
Percolated	110.0 mg.
Dripolated	146.0 mg.
Tea Bags	
Black 5-minute brew	46.0 mg.
Black 1-minute brew	28.0 mg.
Loose Tea	
Black 5-minute brew	40.0 mg.
Green 5-minute brew	35.0 mg.
Cocoa	13.0 mg.
DRUGS	PER PILL
Anacin	32.0 mg.

Drugs	Per Pill
Cafergot	100.0 mg.
Empirin	32.0 mg.
Emprazil	30.0 mg.
Excedrin	65.0 mg.
[Excedrin PM has no caffeine, but does have an antihistamine.]	
Fiorinal	130.0 mg.
Midol	32.4 mg.
Soma Compound	32.0 mg.
Triaminicin	30.0 mg.
Vanquish	33.0 mg.

Caffeine Alternatives

Decaffeinated coffee is *not* the best solution to the caffeine problem. Trichorethylene, which was first used to remove caffeine, was found to cause a high incidence of cancer in test animals. Though the manufacturers have switched to methylene chloride, which is safer, it, too, introduces the same carbon-to-chlorine bond into the body that is characteristic of so many toxic insecticides.

Regular tea is not the answer either, since that has nearly as much caffeine. But herb teas can be quite invigorating, and most natural-food stores have a wide variety to choose from. Then, too, ginseng can give you a real lift, especially Siberian ginseng, much like the one you get from caffeine without the side effects.

Colas, diet or regular, have become as popular as coffee for those to enjoy the caffeine boost. Try substituting club soda or mineral water, or even a flavoured soda if you must. You won't get the caffeine lift, but you'll be doing your body a big favour.

What alcohol Does to Your Body

Alcohol is the most widely used drug in our society, and because it is so available, most people don't think of it as a drug. But it is; and if misused, it can cause a lot of damage to your body.

Alcohol is not a stimulant, but actually a sedative-depressant of the central nervous system.

191

It is capable of rupturing veins.

It does not warm you up, but causes you to feel colder by increasing perspiration and body heat loss.

It destroys brain cells by causing the withdrawal of necessary water from them.

It can deplete the body of vitamin B_1, B_2, B_6, B_{12}, folic acid, vitamin C, vitamin K, zinc, magnesium, and potassium.

Four drinks a day are capable of causing organ damage.

It can hamper the liver's ability to process fat.

What You Drink and When You Drink It

Just because the alcohol content varies in different beverages, don't be fooled. It is true that beer has only about 4 percent alcohol, wine about 12 percent, and whisky up to 50 percent; but a can of beer, a glass of wine, and a shot of whisky all have virtually the identical inebriation potential. In other words, four cans of beer can get you just as tipsy as four shots of tequila.

Surprisingly, what you drink doesn't matter nearly as much as *when* you drink it. Dr. John D. Palmer, of the University of Massachusetts, reports that the length of time alcohol remains circulating in your blood varies throughout the day. Which means, of course, the more time the alcohol spends in your blood, the more time it has to act on your brain cells. Between 2 A.M. and noon are the most vulnerable hours, while later afternoon to early evening are the least. A cocktail at dinner will be burned away 25 percent faster than a Bloody Mary at breakfast. Dr. Palmer has also found that the last drink of a party, consumed after midnight, is metabolised relatively more slowly than the ones that preceded it, and will produce a more lasting rise in blood alcohol.

Vitamins to Decrease Your Taste for Alcohol

Research at the University of Texas by Professor Roger Williams has shown that if alcoholic mice are fed nutritious, vitamin-enriched diets, they quickly lose their interest in alcohol. This seems to hold true for people, since heavy drinkers have been able to break the habit — and even lose interest — with the right

192

diet and proper nutritional supplements. Vitamins A, D, E, C, and all the B vitamins — especially B_{12}, B_6, and B_1 — along with dolomite, choline, inositol, niacin, and a very high-protein diet have brought about the best results. Dr. H.L. Newbold, of New York, who has worked with alcoholics, recommends building up to 5 glutamine capsules [200 mg.] — not glutamic acid — three times a day to control drinking, and working with a good nutritionally orientated doctor for the best all-around regimen.

In experiments done by the veterans Administration, a supplement of tryptophan, given in larger concentrations than occur in a normal diet, has helped alcoholics achieve normal sleeping patterns by reducing or normalising the fragmentation of dreaming [REM]. Because serotonin, a natural tranquiliser substance in the brain has been shown to be reduced in alcoholism, tryptophan can help alcoholics stay dry by relieving some of the symptoms of alcohol-related body chemistry disorders.

XVIII

You and Your Rx

Why Vitamins Have Come Under Attack

The medical establishment considers current therapy to be drugs, surgery, and analysis. Vitamins are rarely used in treatment, and preventive medicine is still in its infancy.

The situation is changing, however, because the public wants health professionals who are knowledgeable about nutrition.

Vitamins are natural substances and therefore not under government control. Many doctors don't like this, because the availability of vitamins can lead to the public's experimenting on its own. Large drugs corporations don't like it because the substances are not patentable, which means they can't make money from them.

There Are Alternatives to Drugs

There are alternatives to drugs which orthomolecular physicians and nutritionally minded individuals are trying before resorting to drugs. Dr. Robert C. Atkins, author of *Dr. Atkins' Diet Revolution*, has his patients try pantothenic acid and about 2,000 mg. of inositol as sleep inducers instead of barbiturate sleeping pills. He has also had success using B_{13} [orotic acid] to lower high blood pressure and B_{15} to control blood sugar.

Before resorting to tranquilisers for your nerves, why not increase your ingestion of goods rich in B, and try a good stress B complex with C two to three times daily and see how you feel?

Garlic, vitamin C, and chicken soup have remarkable natural antibiotic and antihistamine properties.

Instead of becoming dependent upon commercial laxative preparations, why not try bran?

How about switching from commercial antacids to a multiple digestive enzyme?

Vitamins Instead of Valium

Valium, a tranquilliser, is *the* most prescribed drug in the world. Taken for a variety of conditions ranging from simple upsets and insomnia to angina pectoris, it is surely one of the most overused drugs around. [Based on weight it is also the most expensive drug in the world.]

If you're interested in breaking a Valium habit, in finding a nonaddictive natural substitute that will allow you to relax and to sleep, you and your doctor should look into L-tryptophan, an essential amino acid and constituent of all protein foods.

Research at Tufts University and the Sleep Laboratory of the Boston State Hospital has shown that L-tryptophan not only aids in building proteins, but is used by the brain to synthesise the vital brain chemical serotonin — a neuro-transmitter that carries messages between neurons, and one of the biochemical mechanisms of sleep. And that even a 1 g. dose [the tryptophan content

194

of a large meal] can reduce the time it takes to fall asleep and increase time spent sleeping. Also, unlike sleeping medications, tryptophan does not alter the normal stages and cycles of sleep. A tryptophan does not alter the normal stages and cycles of sleep. A tryptophan supplement [2 mg.] should be taken a half hour before bedtime with water or juice [no protein]; a vitamin B_6 [50 mg.] and chelated magnesium [133 mg.]

The Great Medicine Rip-off

More than ever before, people are gulping down drugs, and what they don't realise is that a lot of these medications — prescription as well as over-the-counter — are taking as much as they're giving, at least nutritionally. All too often the drugs either stop the absorption of nutrients or interfere with the cells' ability to use them.

A recent study showed that ingredients found in common over-the-counter cold, pain, and allergy remedies actually lowered the blood level of vitamin A. Since vitamin A protects and strengthens the mucous membranes lining the nose, throat, and lungs, a deficiency could give bacteria a cosy home to multiply in, prolonging the illness the drug was meant to alleviate.

Aspirin, the household wonder drug, the most common ingredient of pain relievers, cold and sinus remedies, is a vitamin-C thief. Even a small amount can *triple* the excretion rate of vitamin C from the body. It can also lead to a deficiency of folic acid, which could cause anaemia as well as digestive disturbances.

Corticosteroids [cortisone, prednisone], used for easing arthritis pain, skin problems, blood and eye disorders, and asthma, have been found to be related to lowered zinc levels.

Laxatives and antacids, taken by millions, have been found to disturb the body's calcium and phosphorus metabolism. And any laxative taken to excess can deplete large amounts of potassium.

Diuretics, commonly prescribed for high blood pressure, and antibiotics are also potassium thieves.

The following is a list of drugs that induce vitamin deficiencies and the vitamins they deplete. Look it over before you take your next medicine.

Three basic mechanisms exist by which drugs induce vitamin deficiencies:

A. Impaired vitamin absorption
B. Impaired vitamin utilisation
C. Enhanced vitamin elimination

A. IMPAIRMENT OF VITAMIN ABSORPTION

Drug	Vitamins depleted
Glutethimide	Folic acid
Cholestyramine	A, D, E, K, and B_{12}
Os-Cal-Mone	B_6
Mineral Oil	A, D, E, and K
Polysporin, Neo-Sporin, Neomycin, Mycolog, Neo-Cortef, Cortisporin, Lidosporin, Mycifradin	K, B_{12}, and folic acid
Kanamycin	K and B_{12}
Tetracycline	K, calcium, magnesium, and iron
Chloramphenical	K
Polymyxin	KSylphonamides
Phazyme	K
Sulphasalazine, Aso-Gantanol	Folic Acid
Colchicine, Colbenemid	B_{12}, A, and potassium
Trifluoperazine	B_{12}
Cortisone	B_6, D, C, zinc, and potassium
Cathartic agents	B_2, K
Antacids	A and B

B. IMPAIRMENT OF VITAMIN UTILISATION

Drug	Vitamins depleted
Coumarins	K
Pro-Banthine, Probital	K
Methotrexate	Folic acid
Triamterene	Folic acid
Pyrimethamine	Folic acid

196

Drug	Vitamins depleted
Trimethoprim	Folic acid
Nitrofurantoin	Folic acid
Phenylbutazone	Folic acid
Aspirin	Folic acid, C, and B_1
Indomethacin	B_1 and C
Bentyl with Phenobarb, Cantil with Phenobarb, Isordil with Phenobarb	K

C. ENHANCED VITAMIN EXCRETION

Drug	Vitamins depleted
Aldactazide, Altactone	Potassium
Isoniazid	B_6
Hydralazine	B_6
Ser-Ap-Es	B_6
Penicillamine	B_6
Chlorothiazide	Magnesium and potassium
Boric Acid	B_2
Bronkotabs, Bronkolixer	K
Chardonna	K

DRUGS WITH MULTIPLE MECHANISMS

Drug	Vitamins depleted
Diethylstilbestrol	B_6
Anticonvulsants	Folic acid and D
Phenytoin	Folic acid and D
Barbiturates	Folic acid and D
Oral contraceptive steroids	Folic acid, C, and B_6
Alcohol	B_1, folic acid, and K
Betapar	B_6, C, zinc, and potassium

XIX

Losing It —Diets by the Pound

First keep in mind the dangers of too much sugar and salt. And, in case you don't think you eat too much sugar and salt let me remind you of the "invisible" sugar and salt you can be taking.

Kinds of Sugars

More than a hundred substances that qualify as sweet can be called sugars. The ones we come in contact with most often are *fructose*, a natural sugar found in fruit and honey; *glucose*, the body's blood sugar and the simplest form of sugar in which a carbohydrate is assimilated; *dextrose*, made from cornstarch and chemically identical to glucose; *lactose*, milk sugar, *maltose*, the sugar formed from the starch by the action of yeast: and *sucrose*, the sugar that is obtained from sugar cane or beets and refined to the product that reaches us as granules.

Brown sugar, which many people assume to be healthier than white sugar, is merely sugar crystals coated with molasses syrup. Honey is a blend of fructose and glucose. And then there are the various corn sweeteners, derived from cornstarch and composed mainly of dextrose, maltose, and the more complex sugars.

Dangers of Too Much Sugar

The big problem with sugar is that we eat too much of it (over 154 pounds [300 teaspoons] per person in 1984) and often don't even know it. All carbohydrate sweeteners qualify as sugar, even though they may be called by other names; and when sucrose is the number-three ingredient on a box of cereal, corn syrup number five, and honey number seven, you don't realize it but you're eating something that is 50 percent sugar!

The consumer today is hooked on sugar right from the start. Baby formulas are sweetened with sugar, as are many baby foods. Because sugar also acts as a preservative, retains and absorbs moisture, it's often in products we never think of as containing it, products such as salt, peanut butter, canned vegetables, bouillon cubes, and more. Would you believe that the ketchup you put on your hamburger has just less than 8 percent more sugar than ice cream? That cream substitute for coffee is 65 percent sugar compared to 51 percent for a chocolate bar?

The fact is, we're eating too much sugar for our health. It is beyond argument that sugar is a prime factor in tooth decay. Also, one-third of our population is overweight, and obesity increases the possibility of heart disease, diabetes, hypertension, gallstones, back problems, and arthritis. Not that sugar alone is the cause, but its presence in foods induces you to eat more, and if you cut your calorie count without cutting your sugar intake, you'll lose nutrients faster than pounds. Sugar is also the villain where hypoglycemia is concerned, and, though there have been arguments pro and con, directly or indirectly a factor in diabetes and heart disease.

How Sweet It Is

Hidden sugars are where you least expect them. If you want to be a sugar detective, my advice is to check labels. Look for sucrose substitutes such as corn syrup or corn sugar, and watch out for words ending in "-ose," which indicates the presence of sugar. A sugar by any name is still a sugar. And remember that not even medicines are immune from added sweeteners!

Dangers of Too Much Salt

Taking things with a grain of salt is all well and good, but eating things with it might be a different story. The normal intake of sodium chloride (table salt) is 6 to 18 g. daily, but an intake over 14 g. is considered excessive. And too many of us are being excessive. The average American consumes about 15 pounds (a bowling ball) of salt each year!

Too much salt can cause hypertension (high blood pressure), which increases the chances of heart disease, and has recently been cited as one of the causes for migraine headaches. It causes abnormal fluid retention, which can result in dizziness and swelling of the legs. Also it may cause potassium to be lost in the urine. And in addition, too much salt can harm you nutritionally by interfering with the proper utilization of protein foods.

High-Salt Traps

Just because you stay away from pretzels and snack foods and don't pour on the table salt doesn't mean you're not getting more salt than you should. Salt traps are as hidden from view as sugar ones.

If you want to keep your salt intake down:

> Hold back on beer. (There's 25 mg. sodium in every 12 ounces.)
>
> Avoid the use of baking soda, monosodium glutamate (MSG, Accent), and baking powder in food preparation.
>
> Stay away from laxatives, most of which contain sodium.
>
> Do not drink or cook with water treated by a home water softener; it adds sodium to the water.
>
> Look for the words SALT, SODIUM, or the chemical symbol *Na* when reading foods labels.
>
> Don't eat cured meat such as ham, bacon, corned beef, or frankfurters, sausage, shellfish, any canned or frozen meat, poultry, or fish to which sodium has been added.
>
> When dining out, ask for an inside cut of meat, or chops or steaks without added salt.
>
> Watch out for diet sodas — the calories might be low, but the sodium content is *high*!

Mindell Dieting Tips

Before starting any diet, check with your physician. If you don't feel that your family doctor understands your dieting needs, contact a bariatrician, who specialises in the field.

If you're on a low- or no-carbohydrate diet, beware of artificially sweetened "sugarless" or "dietetic" gum or candy that has sorbitols, mannitols, or hexitols. These ingredients are metabolised in the system as carbohydrates, only more slowly.

If you're on a diet that allows alcohol, a glass of wine before dinner stimulates the gastric juices and aids in proper digestion.

Watch out for such diet fallacies as:

Gelatin dessert is nonfattening.
Grapefruit causes you to lose weight.
Fruits have no calories.
High-protein foods have no calories.
A pound of steak is not as fattening as a potato.
Toast has much fewer calories than bread.

Whatever you're eating, sit down to eat it, and eat it slowly. [You might expend more calories standing than sitting, but you tend to eat more that way, too.]

When selecting fruit, remember that all fruits are not equal, that an apple, a banana, or a pear has more calories and carbohydrates than half a melon, a cup of raw strawberries, or a fresh tangerine.

When choosing your vegetable, take green beans instead of peas [you save 41 calories on a half-cup serving], spinach instead of mixed vegetables [you save 35 calories], and mashed potatoes — if you must — instead of fried potatoes [you save 139 calories].

Carbohydrate watchers, don't underestimate onions; one cup of cooked onions has 18g.

If you're counting every calorie, realise that 1 tablespoon of lecithin granules contains 50 calories and a lecithin capsule about 68.

Try a one-day-a-week fast [the ancient Greeks did it]. Limit yourself to cold tap water [not iced] or herb tea with lemon or lime juice. Nothing else. This should pep you up, too.

Mindell Vitamin-balanced Diet to Lose and Live By

I know your mother told it to you, but it is true anyway — breakfast *is* the most important meal of the day. It comes after the longest period of time that you've been without food, and

201

you cannot catch up nutritionally by eating a good lunch or dinner later.

If you're dieting, it is especially important to perk up your energy level at the start of the day. Even if you're in a hurry. And since most people I know are rushed in the morning, I advise the following blender breakfast.

BREAKFAST

8 oz nonfat or low-fat milk [or juice]
A flavoured low-calorie protein powder that contains nutritional
    yeast, lecithin, and fructose
4 ice cubes
Mix well in blender for 60 seconds. Calories, approximately: 150

This mixture can be frozen and used as a dessert for dinner or a pick-me-up snack if your calorie quotient allows.

Lunch is a tricky meal. Fast-food restaurants are seductively convenient, and nothing blows a diet faster than "a few French fries" and a "tiny milkshake". If you really want to lose weight, think more along these lines:

LUNCH

Monday, Wednesday, Saturday, and Sunday

A modest portion [3–5 ounces] of water-packed canned or fresh fish, a large raw vegetable salad [with lemon or vinegar dressing], and a piece of fruit.

Tuesday, Thursday, and Friday

2 eggs [prepared without fat] or cottage or pot cheese [no more than 1 cup], raw vegetables, 1 slice of bread with a light coating of margerine, and a fruit for dessert. [The American Heart Association suggests only 3 whole eggs per week, though many doctors allow more. Check with your own physician.]

Dinner is usually a dieter's downfall, but it doesn't have to be that way:

DINNER

Five nights a week you should have fish [sole, trout, salmon, halibut, etc.] or poultry broiled, boiled, or roasted [remove skin before eating poultry]; and two nights a week you can have meat; once again broiled, boiled, or roasted; a cooked vegetable, a large salad [no more than 1 teaspoon oil in the dressing], a small boiled or baked potato once or twice a week, and a fresh fruit for dessert.

Stay away from alcohol — try sparkling mineral water with lime instead. As for other beverages, herb teas and plain old water are best.

Take your supplements six days a week and rest on the seventh. By doing this, you'll never have to worry about a build-up of fat-soluble vitamins in the system.

SUPPLEMENTS

Time-release multiple vitamin with chelated minerals [at least 50 mg. B_1, B_2, and B_6 per tablet] taken A.M. and P.M.
Time-release vitamin C, 1,000 mg. with rose hips bioflavonoids, 2 tablets taken A.M. and P.M.

A multiple chelated mineral tablet with at least 500 mg. calcium and 250 mg. magnesium per tablet [must also have manganese, zinc, iron, selenium, chromium, copper, iodine, and potassium] taken A.M. and P.M.

Dry vitamin E, 400 IU — D-alpha-tocopherol with selenium, chromium, vitamin C, and ascorbates taken A.M. and P.M.

RNA 100 mg. — DNA 100 mg., 3 tablets daily, 6 days a week.

Lecithin, 1,200 mg. [6 capsules] daily. [If you use lecithin granules in breakfast drink, this supplement is not necessary.]

Vitamin B_{15}, 50 mg. in the A.M.

PART FOUR

LOOKING YOUR BEST FROM THE INSIDE OUT

XX

Staying Beautiful — Staying Handsome

Vitamins for Healthy Skin

What you look like on the outside depends a lot on what you do for yourself on the inside. And as far as you skin is concerned, vitamins and proper nutrition are essential.

To look your best, make sure you're getting 55 to 65 g. of protein a day. Drink eight glasses of water daily [herbal teas can count for a few of them], and keep your milk and yoghurt consumption restricted to the nonfat variety. Keep away from chocolate, nuts, dried fruids, fried foods, cola drinks, coffee, alcohol, cigarettes, and excessive salt. Also, do not use sugar. Small amounts of honey or blackstrap molasses will sweeten just as well and you'll look better for it.

A good start toward healthy, glowing skin is a daily protein drink. It can be taken in place of any meal, but it makes an especially good breakfast.

PROTEIN DRINK

6 oz. raw nonfat milk
1 tbsp. nutritional yeast powder [lots of B vitamins]
3 tbsp, acidophilus [promotes friendly bacteria]
1 tbsp, granulated lecithin [breaks down bumps or cholesterol under the skin]
2 tbsp. protein powder
½–1 tbsp. blackstrap molasses or honey
Carob powder, bananas, strawberries, or any fresh fruit for flavouring
Mix in blender. [Add 3–4 ice cubes, if desired.]

Multiple-vitamin and mineral complex — 1 daily
Take after any meal. Important for skin tone and nerve health.

B complex, 100 mg. [time release] — 1 daily

Take after any meal. B_2 [riboflavin] and B_6 [pyridoxine] reduce facial oiliness and blackhead formation.

Vitamin A [dry form], 25,000 IU — 2 daily for 6 days a week

Take 1 after breakfast and 1 after dinner.

Maintains soft, smooth, disease-free skin.

Builds resistance to infections.

Rose hips vitamin C, 500 mg. with bioflavonoids — 4 daily

Take 1 after each meal and at bedtime. Aids in preventing the spread of acne. Promotes healing of wounds, bruising, and scar tissue. Helps to prevent breakage of capillaries on face.

Vitamin E, 400 IU [dry form] — 3 daily

Take 1 after each meal. Improves circulation in tiny face capillaries. Aids in healing by replacing cells on the skin's outer layers. Works with vitamin C in making skin less suceptible to acne. Use vitamin-E oil externally on skin for healing butns, abrasions, and scar tissue.

Multiple chelated minerals — 6 daily

Take 2 tablets after each meal [or 3 in A.M. and P.M.] Helps maintain the acid-alkaline balance of the blood necessary for a clear complexion. Calcium is for soft, smooth skin tissue; copper for skin colour; iron to improve pale skin; potassium for dry skin and acne; zinc for external and internal wound healing.

Choline and inositol, 1,000 mg. — 4 tablets daily.

Take 2 after breakfast and dinner. [Lecithin granules, 2 tbsp. daily, can be substituted for choline and inositol tabs.] Helps emulsify cholesterol [fatty deposits or bumps under the skin]. Purifies the kidneys which aids the skin.

Acidophilus — 6 tbsp. daily

Take 2 tbsp. or 6 capsules after each meal. Helps fight skin eruptions caused by unfriendly bacteria in the system.

Chlorophyll — 3 tsp. or 9 tablets daily

Take 1 tsp. or 3 tablets after each meal. Reduces hazard of bacterial contamination. Possesses antibiotic action. An excellent aid to wound healing, after washing thoroughly with a soap substitute made from the comfrey plant.

If the face is badly blemished, extra zinc is advised. Take six tablets daily, two after each meal. Aids in growth and repair of injured tissues.

Vitamins for Healthy Hair

Shampoos and conditioners are not enough. To make sure that you're giving your crowning glory its due, you have to be aware that nutrition plays a very important role in having terrific, shiny hair. Unlike the skin, hair cannot repair itself; but you *can* get new, healthier hair to grow.

The first thing to do is examine your diet. Does it include fish, wheat germ, yeast, and liver? It should. The vitamins and minerals that these foods supply are what your hair needs, along with frequent scalp massage, a good pH-balanced, protein-enriched shampoo, and supplements.

SUPPLEMENTS

Multiple-vitamin and mineral complex — 1 daily
Take after any meal. Important for general health of hair.
B complex, 100 mg. [time release] — 1 daily
Take after any meal. B vitamins are essential for hair growth. Adelle Davis found that pantothenic acid, folic acid, and PABA helped restore grey hair to its natural colour.
Vitamin A, 25,000 IU — 1–2 daily 6 days a week
Take A.M. and P.M. Works with vitamin B to keep hair shiny.
Multiple chelated minerals — 1 daily
Take with breakfast. Minerals such as silicon, sulphur, iodine, and iron help prevent falling hair.

Keep in mind that you need some fatty acids, vitamin E, and choline in your body for vitamin A to survive.

Vitamins for Hands and Feet

Your hands take lots of abuse. Detergents strip away natural oils, and water and weather alone can cause chapping. Rubber gloves are a good idea, but if you already have splits in your skin or some sort of dermatitis, they should *not* be put directly on your hands. [A pair of cotton gloves beneath the rubber ones will absorb perspiration and prevent reinfection.] Also, do not use cornstarch in the gloves; it can promote the growth of micororganisms. If you want to use something to absorb the moisture, try plain, unscented talcum powder.

As for toenails and fingernails, the best remedy for problems is diet. Gelatin is commonly accepted as the cure for weak nails, but this is a misconception. The nails do need protein, but gelatin is a poor supplier. Not only are two essential amino acids missing, but another amino acid, glycine, is supplied in amounts you do not need. Foods rich in sulphur, such as egg yolks, should be part of your diet, and desiccated liver [powder or tablets] should be taken as a supplement.

SUPPLEMENTS

Multiple-vitamin and mineral complex — 1 daily
  Take after any meal. Promotes general skin health and growth of nails.
B Complex, 100 mg. [time release] — 1 daily
  Take after any meal. Helps build resistance to fungus infections and vital to nail growth.
Vitamin A, 25,000 IU — 1 daily 6 days a week
  Take after any meal. Helps to prevent splitting nails.
Vitamin E, 100–400 IU — 1–2 daily
  Take in A.M. and P.M. Necessary for proper utilisation of vitamin A.
Multiple chelated minerals — 1 daily
  Take after any meal. Iron helps strengthen brittle nails, zinc gets rid of white spots.

Natural Cosmetics — What's in Them

Many cosmetics nowadays are advertised as "natural," but looking at the ingredients can cause you to wonder. To be sure of what you're getting, read the label carefully. The following explanations of cosmetic ingredients should make things clearer.

Amyl Dimethyl PABA — a sunscreening agent from PABA, a
  B-complex factor.

Annatto — a vegetable colour obtained from the seeds of a tropical plant.

Avocado oil — a vegetable oil obtained from avocados

Caprylic/Capric triglyceride — an emollient obtained from coconut oil

Carrageenan — a natural thickening agent from dried Irish moss

Castor oil — an emollient oil collected from the pressing of castor bean seeds

Cetyl alcohol — a component of vegetable oils

Cetyl palmitate — a component of palm and coconut oils

Citric acid — a natural organic acid found widely in citrus plants

Cocamide DEA — a thickener obtained from coconut oil

Coconut oil — obtained by pressing the kernels of the seeds of the coconut palm

Decyl oleate — obtained from tallow or coconut oil

Disodium monolaneth-5-sulphosuccinate — obtained from lanolin and used to improve the texture of hair

Fragrance — oils obtained from flowers, grasses, roots, and stems that give off a pleasant or agreeable odour

Goat milk whey — protein-rich whey obtained from goat's milk

Glyceryl stearate — an organic emulsifier obtained from glycerin

Hydrogenated castor oil — a waxy material obtained from castor oil

Imidzaolidinyl urea — a preservative derived naturally as a product of protein metabolism [hydrolysis]

Lanolin alcohol — a constituent of lanolin that performs as an emollient and emulsifier

Laureth-3 — an organic material obtained from coconut and palm oils

Methyl glucoside sesquistearate – an organic emulsifier obtained from a natural simple sugar

Mineral oil — an organic emollient and lubricant

Olive oil — a natural oil obtained from olives

Peanut oil — a vegetable oil obtained from peanuts

Pectin —derived from citrus fruits and apple peel

PEG lanolin — an emollient and emulsifier obtained from lanolin

Petrolatum — petroleum jelly

P.O.E. [20] methyl glucoside sesquistearate — an organic

emulsifier from a simple natural sugar

Potassium sorbate — obtained from sorbic acid found in the berries of mountain ash

Safflower oil-hybrid — a natural emollient obtained from a strain of specially cultivated plants

Sesame oil — oil of pressed sesame seeds

Sodium cetyl sulphate — a detergent and emulsifier obtained from coconut oil

Sodium laureth sulphate — a detergent obtained from coconut oil

Sodium lauryl sulphate — a detergent obtained from coconut oil

Sodium PCA — a natural-occurring humectant found in the skin where it acts as the natural moisturiser

Sorbic acid — a natural preservative derived from berries of mountain ash

Tocopherol — a natural vitamin E

Undecylenamide DEA — a natural preservative derived from castor oil

Water — the universal solvent, and the major constituent of all living material

XXI

Staying Young, Energetic, and Sexy

Retarding the Aging Process Through the Remarkable Nucleic Acids

Aging is caused by the degeneration of cells. Our bodies are made up of millions of these cells, each with a life of somewhere around two years or less. But before a cell dies, it reproduces itself. Why, then, you might wonder, shouldn't we look the same now as we did ten years ago? The reason for this is that with each successive reproduction, the cell goes through some alteration — basically, deterioration. So as our cells change, deteriorate, we grow old.

Dr. Benjamin S. Frank, author of *Nucleic Acid Therapy in Aging and Degenerative Disease* [New York: Psychological Library, 1969; revised 1974], has found that deteriorating cells can be rejuvenated if provided with substances that directly nourish them — substances such as nucleic acids.

DNA [deoxyribonucleic acid] and RNA [ribonucleic acid] are our nucleic acids. DNA is essentially a chemical boiler-plate for new cells. It sends out RNA molecules like a team of well-trained workers to form them. When DNA stops giving the orders to RNA, new cell construction ceases — as does life. But by helping the body stay well supplied with nucleic acids, Dr. Frank has found that you can look and feel six to twelve years younger than you actually are.

According to Dr. Frank, we need 1 to 1½ g. of nucleic acid daily. Though the body can produce its own nucleic acids, he feels they are broken down too quickly into less useful compounds and should be supplied from external sources if the aging process is to be retarded, even reversed.

Foods rich in nucleic acids are wheat germ, bran, spinach, asparagus, mushrooms, fish [especially sardines, salmon, and anchovies], chicken liver, oatmeal, and onions. He recommends a diet where seafood is eaten seven times a week, along with two glasses of skimmed milk, a glass of fruit or vegetable juice, and four glasses of water daily.

After only two months of RNA–DNA supplementation and diet, Dr. Frank found that his patients had more energy and that there was a substantial diminution of lines and wrinkles, with healthier, rosier, and younger-looking skin in evidence.

One of the most recent arrivals in the battle to combat aging is SOD (superoxide dismutase). This enzyme fortifies the body against the ravages of free racdials, destructive molecules which speed the aging process by destroying healthy cells as well as attacking collagen ("cement" that holds cells together).

As we age, our bodies produce less SOD, so supplementation

213

— along with a natural diet that restricts free radical formation — can help increase our energetic and productive years. It's important to note, though, that SOD can become inactive very quickly if essential minerals, such as zinc, copper, and manganese, are not supplied.

DHEA (dehydroepiandrosterone), a natural hormone that is produced by the adrenal glands, is now also being used in anti-aging regimens, since one of its properties is that it can "de-excite" the body's processes and thereby slow down the production of fats, hormones, and acids that contribute to aging.

Basic Vitamin-Mineral RNA–DNA Programme

Along with proper diet, a good supplement regimen is important to the success of an RNA–DNA programme. I've found that the following works best:

High.potency multiple vitamin with chelated minerals [time release preferred] A.M. and P.M.
Vitamin C, 1,000 mg. with bioflavonoids, A.M. and P.M.
Vitamin E, 400 IU [dry form] with antioxidants A.M. and P.M.
RNA–DNA, 100-mg. tablets, 1 daily for one month, then 2 daily
    for the next month, then 3 daily thereafter, 6 days a week
Stress B complex A.M. and P.M.

High-Pep Energy Regimen

Whether you want to feel good, or just look good, exercise, diet, and the right supplements are the tickets to high energy.

If you're not into jogging, can't afford the sneakers, don't play tennis, find yourself reluctant to swim in twenty-below weather, and hate calisthenics, I have the perfect exercise for you — jumping rope.

A jump rope is inexpensive, convenient [you can take it everywhere], and lots of fun to use. And it works! In terms of calories burned, jumping rope can outdo bicycling, tennis and swimming. An average person of about 150 pounds uses up 720 calories an hour jumping rope [120 to 140 turns per minute]. When you realise that an hour of tennis uses up only 420 calories, you have a better idea of just how good jumping rope can be for you.

For keeping energy high, remember to eat a combination of two protein foods [or a protein drink], at each meal; drink at least six glasses of water daily [a half hour before or after meals]; avoid refined sugar, flour, tobacco, alcohol, tea, coffee, soft drinks, processed and fried foods.

A good pep-up protein drink:

2 tbsp. protein powder
1 tbsp. lecithin powder
2 tbsp. acidophilus liquid
1 tbsp. nutritional yeast
1 tbsp. safflower oil [optional]

Blend with milk, water, or juice in blender for 1 minute.

High-Pep Supplements

With breakfast:

High-potency multiple vitamin with chelated minerals [time release preferred]
2 stress B complex with C
Vitamin E, 400 IU
High-potency multiple chelated mineral
Acidophilus, 3 capsules or 2 tbsp. liquid
Lecithin powder, 1 tbsp. or 3 19-g. capsules
3 calcium and magnesium tablets

With lunch:

2 stress B complex with C
Vitamin E, 400 IU
Acidophilus, 3 capsules or 2 tbsp. liquid
Lecithin powder, 1 tbsp. or 3 19-g. capsules
Optional: vitamin B_{12}, liver tablets, digestive enzymes

With dinner:

2 stress B complex with C
Vitamin E, 400 IU
Acidophilus, 3 capsules or 2 tbsp. liquid

Lecithin powder, 1 tbsp. or 3 19-g. capsules
Optional: digestive enzymes

Vitamins and Sex

The important thing to remember is that if you're not feeling up to par your sex drive is going to suffer along with the rest of you.

There have been many claims for vitamin E in relationship to sex. Studies have indeed shown that it increases the fertility in males and females and helps restore male potency. That it strongly influences the sex drive in men and women has yet to be proven, though I have met many vitamin-E takers who are happily convinced that it does.

Another noteworthy sex nutrient is zinc. The largest percentage of zinc in a man's body is found in the prostate, and a lack of the mineral can produce testicular atrophy and prostate trouble. [See page 92.]

Remember, vitamins that keep up your energy levels will also do a lot for your sexual performance.

Food and Supplements for Better Sex

Oysters [yes, they're high in zinc], shellfish of all kinds, brewer's yeast, wheat bran, wheat germ, whole grains, and pumpkin seeds. Incorporating these foods in a programme that includes a high-protein and basically low-carbohydrate diet, exercise, and supplements is as good as an aphrodisiac for lovers.

SUPPLEMENTS

nsp [see page 119]
Vitamin B complex, 50 mg., 1–3 times daily
Vitamin E, 400 Iu, 1–3 times daily
Zinc, 50 mg. [chelated], 1–3 times daily
Ginseng 500 mg. 3 times daily 1 hour before meals

Although a lot is still going to depend on the male involved, I believe that octacosanol (which is a natural food substance present in very small amounts in many vegetable oils, the leaves of alfalfa and wheat, wheat germ, and other foods) has an energy-releasing function, increasing strength and stamina, and in laboratory experiments it seems to improve reproductive disturbances.

If you try it, don't be impatient, it often takes 4 to 6 weeks for beneficial effects from octacosanol to be noticed.

Always keep in mind, too, that an energizing diet of raw or lightly cooked foods, rich in B vitamins and amino acids, will contribute to a good sex life.

XXII

Travelling Healthy

Vitamins On the Go

Don't forget to pack the vitamins! Believe it or not, vitamins on vacation — or whatever your reason for travelling — are as important as they are at home. In many cases even more so. The stresses of travel, though they often go unnoticed, can be significant.

If you're travelling to warm or tropical places, be sure that the vitamins you take are in opaque containers and that you keep them in a cool place, not out in the sun. Pack a good sunscreening cream with PABA or a vitamin-E preparation [20,000 IU]. If you have been taking vitamin-D supplements and want to get off for a while, this is the time. A wise choice of vitamins to bring along would be:

High potency multiple vitamin and minerals [take 1 with breakfast and dinner]
Vitamin E, 400 IU [dry form] [take 1–2 daily]
Vitamin C, 1,000 mg. with bioflavonoids [take with breakfast and dinner]
Stress B complex, 50 mg. [take 2–3 times daily]

If you're heading to chillier environs, be sure to take plenty of vitamin C [time release recommended], and if you plan to be indoors a lot, vitamin D also. The vitamins listed above will work in any climate, but if you do find yourself in an area colder than you're used to, remember to take the vitamin C with all your meals instead of just breakfast and dinner.

Acidophilus can be a traveller's best friend. If you're travelling to foreign ports, keep in mind that acidophilus [3 capsules or 2 tablespoons liquid] three times a day is good for diarrhoea prevention.

Are Foreign Vitamins Different?

Vitamins the world over are the same, only dosages vary. Read the label. The metric system is used internationally for measurement, and nutrients are measured by weight. In the metric system, the energy value of food is measured in units called *joules*, or kilocalories, better known as calories. Four of our calories are the equivalent of 17 joules. In other words, a joule is slightly more than four times a calorie.

XXIII

Vitamin Cautions

Cautions

Though we all know that vitamins are good for us, there are times, situations, and metabolic conditions where caution and special adjustment are advised. I recommend you look over the following list carefully for your own well-being and in order to get the most from your vitamins.

– Chronic hypervitaminosis A can occur in patients receiving megadoses as treatment for dermatological conditions.

218

- A deficiency of vitamin A can lead to loss of vitamin C.
- An oversupply of vitamin B_1 (thiamine) can affect thyroid and insulin production and might cause B_6 deficiency, as well as loss of other B vitamins.
- Prolonged ingestion of any B vitamin can result in significant depletion of the others.
- Pregnant women should check with their doctors before taking sustained doses of over 50 mg. of vitamin B_6 (pyridoxine).
- B_6 should not be taken by anyone under L-dopa treatment for Parkinson's disease.
- Large doses of vitamin B_2 (riboflavin), especially if taken without antioxidant supplements, may cause a sensitivity to sunlight.
- Because vitamin D promotes absorption of calcium, a large excess of stored vitamin D can cause too much calcium in the blood (hypercalcaemia).
- Don't eat raw egg whites. They deactivate the body's biotin.
- It is possible that large amounts of vitamin C might reverse the anticoagulant activity of the blood thinner warfarin, commonly prescribed as the drug Coumadin.
- Diabetes and heart patients should check with their doctors, because vitamin C might necessitate a lower dosage of pills.
- Megadoses of vitamin C wash out B_{12} and folic acid, so be sure you are taking at least the daily requirement of both.
- Excessive doses of choline, taken over a long period of time, may produce a deficiency of vitamin B_6.
- If you have a heart disorder, check with your physician for the proper vitamin-D dosage to take.
- Vitamin E should be used cautiously by anyone with an overactive thyroid, diabetes, high blood pressure, or rheumatic heart disease. (If you have any of these conditions, start at a very low dosage and build up gradually by 100 IU daily each month to between 400 and 800 IU.)
- Rheumatic heart fever sufferers should know that they have an imbalance between the two sides of their hearts and large vitamin-E dosages can increase the imbalance and worsen

the condition. (Before using supplements, consult your physician.)

- Vitamin E can elevate blood pressure in hypertensives, but if supplementation is started with a low dosage and increased slowly, the end result will be an eventual lowering of the pressure through the vitamin's diuretic properties. Diabetics have been able to reduce their insulin levels with E. Check with your physician.
- Decreases in vitamin E should be gradual, too.
- An excessive intake of folic acid can mask symptoms of pernicious anaemia.
- High doses of folic acid for extended periods of time are not recommended for anyone with a medical history of convulsive disorders or hormone-related cancer.
- Folic acid and PABA might inhibit the effectiveness of sulfonamides, such as Gantrisin.
- Megadoses of vitamin K can build up and cause a red cell breakdown and artaemia.
- Patients on the blood thinner Dicumarol should be aware that synthetic K could counteract the effectiveness of the drug. Conversely, the drug inhibits the absorption of natural vitamin K.
- Sweats and flushes can occur from too much vitamin K.
- Niacin should be used cautiously by anyone with severe diabetes, glaucoma, peptic ulcers, or with impaired liver function.
- Do not give niacin to your dog or cat; it causes flushing and sweating and greatly discomforts the animal. Do not supplement a pet's diet with vitamins A or D unless your vet specifically advises it.
- Excessive amounts of PABA (Para-aminobenzoic acid) in certain individuals can have a negative effect on the liver, kidneys, and heart.
- Iron should not be taken by anyone with sickle-cell anaemia, haemochromatosis, or thalassaemia.
- If your iron supplement is ferrous sulphate, you're losing vitamin E.
- Large quantities of caffeine can inhibit iron absorption.
- Anyone with kidney malfunction should not take more

than 3,000 mg. of magnesium on a daily basis.

- Too much manganese will reduce utilization of the body's iron.
- High doses of manganese can cause motor difficulties and weakness in certain individuals.
- Diets high in fat increase phosphorus absorption and lower your calcium levels.
- If you take cortisone and aldosterone drugs, such as Aldactone and prednisone, you lose potassium and retain sodium. Check with your physician for proper supplements.
- Excessive perspiration can cause a depletion of sodium.
- Too much sodium can cause a potassium loss.
- Excessive zinc intakes can result in iron and copper losses.
- If you add zinc to your diet, be sure you're getting enough vitamin A.
- Anyone suffering from Wilson's disease is susceptible to copper toxicity.
- Too much cobalt may cause an unwanted enlargement of the thyroid gland.
- Anyone taking thyroid medication should be aware that kelp also affects that gland. If you have been using both, a consultation with your doctor and retesting are advised. You might need *less* prescription medicine than you think.
- Large amounts of raw cabbage can cause an iodine deficiency and throw off thyroid production in individuals with existing low-iodine intakes.
- Milk that contains synthetic vitamin D can deplete the body of magnesium.
- Heavy coffee and tea drinkers — cola drinkers, too — should be aware that large caffeine ingestion creates an inositol shortage.
- Inform your doctor if you're taking large amounts of vitamin C. C can change results of lab tests for sugar in the blood and urine and give false negative results in tests for blood in stool specimens.
- Don't engage in strenuous physical activity within four hours after taking vitamin A if you want optimum absorption.

- Copper has a tendency to accumulate in the blood and deplete the brain's zinc supplies.
- Tryptophan should not be taken with protein; use juice or water to swallow tablets, not milk.
- RNA–DNA supplements increase serum uric acid levels and should *not* be taken by anyone with gout.
- Tyrosine and phenylalanine may increase blood pressure and should *not* be taken with MAO inhibitors or other antidepressant drugs. These amino acids are also contraindicated for anyone with pigmented malignant melanomas.
- PABA is contraindicated with *methotrexate* (MEXATE), a cancer-fighting drug.
- Folacin (folic acid) decreases the anticonvulsant action of *phenytoin* (DILANTIN).
- Antibiotics are reduced in their effectiveness when taken with supplements. (Take supplements at least an hour before or two hours after prescription antibiotics.)
- Calcium can interfere with the effectiveness of tetracycline.
- High doses of vitamin D or calcium ascorbate are contraindicated if you are taking the heart medication *digoxin* LANOXIN).
- Broad spectrum antibiotics should not be taken with high doses of vitamin A.
- Vitamin A should not be taken in conjunction with the acne drug ACCUTANE (*isotretinoin*).
- Choline is not recommended during the depressive phase of manic-depressive conditions, since it can deepen this particular sort of depression.
- Papaya, as well as raw pineapple, is not recommended for anyone with an ulcer.

BIBLIOGRAPHY

I owe a great debt of thanks to the many scientists, doctors, nutritionists, professors, and researchers whose painstaking and all too often unrewarding work in the field of vitamins and nutrition has made this book possible.

The following is given to show my sincere appreciation and make known the foundation upon which I have built my knowledge. Many of the books are highly technical and confusing for the layman, meant as they are for professionals in the field. But others, which I have marked with an asterisk, I heartily recommend to you for further reading and a healthier future.

*Abrahamson, E.M., and Pezet, A.W. *Body, Mind and Sugar*. New York: Holt, Rinehart and Winston, 1951.
*Adams, Ruth. *The Complete Home Guide to All the Vitamins*. New York: Larchmont Books, 1972.
*Adams, Ruth, and Murray, Frank. *Minerals: Kill or Cure*. New York: Larchmont Books, 1976.
*Aguilar, Nona. *Totally Natural Beauty*. New York: Rawson Associates Publishers, 1977.
*Airola, Paavo. *Are You Confused?* Phoenix, AZ: Health Plus, 1972.
*———. *How to Get Well*. Phoenix, AZ: Health Plus, 1975.
*———. *Hypoglycaemia. A Better Approach*. Phoenix, AZ: Health Plus, 1977.
Amberson, Rosanne. *Raising Your Cat*. New York: Bonanza Books, 1979.
*Atkins, Robert C. *Dr. Atkins' Diet Revolution*. New York: David McKay, 1972.
*Bailey, Hubert. *Vitamin E: Your Key to a Healthy Heart*. New York: ARC Books, 1964, 1966.
Bieri, John G. "Fat-soluble vitamins in the eighth revision of the Recommended Dietary Allowances." *Journal of the American Dietetic Association* 64 [February 1974).
Blood: The River of Life. American National Red Cross, 1976.
*Borsaak, Henry. *Vitamins: What They Are and How They Can Benefit You*. New York: Pyramid Books, 1971.
"Bread: You can't Judge a Loaf by Its Color." *Consumer Reports* 41 [May 1976].

*Bricklin, Mark. *Practical Enxyclopedia of Natural Healing*. Emmaus, PA: Rodale Press, 1976.

Brody, Jane E. "Cancer-blocking Agents Found in Foods." *The New York Times*, 6 March 1979.

*Burack, Richard, with Fox, Fred J. *New Handbook of Prescription Drugs*. New York: Pantheon Books, 1967.

Burton, Benjamin. *Human Nutrition*. 3rd ed. New York: McGraw-Hill, 1976. "Buying Beef." *Consumer Reports* 39 [September 1974].

*Carr, William H.A. *The Basic Book of the Cat*. New York: Gramercy Publishing Co., 1963.

*Chapman, Esther. *How to Use the 12 Tissue Salts*. New York: Pyramid Books, 1977.

*Clark, Linda, *The Best of Linda Clark*. New Canaan, CT: Keats Publishing Co., 1976.

*——. *Know Your Nutrition*. New Canaan, CT: Keats Publishing Co., 1973.

*——. *Secrets of Health and Beauty*. New York: Jove Publications, 1977.

*Consumer Reports, Editors of. *The Medicine Show*. Mount Vernon, NY: Consumers Union, 1961.

Copper, Barber, Mitchell, Rynberge, Green. *Nutrition in Health and Disease*. New York: Lippincott, 1963.

Cumulative Index for Journal of Applied Nutrition. La Habra, CA: International College of Applied Nutrition, 1947–76, 1976.

*Davis, Adelle. *Let's Eat Right to Keep Fit*. New York: Harcourt, Brace and World, 1954.

*——. *Let's Get Well*. New York: Harcourt, Brace and World, 1965.

*——. *Let's have Healthy Children*. 2nd. ed. New York: Harcourt, Brace and World, 1959.

*Dufty, William, *Sugar Blues*. Pennsylvania: Chilton Book Co., 1975.

*Ebon, Martin. *Which Vitamins Do You Need?* New York: Bantam Books, 1974.

Flynn, Margaret A. "The Cholesterol Controversy." *Journal of the American Pharmacy* NS18 [May 1978].

"Food Facts Talk Back." *Journal of the American Dietetic Association*, 1977.

*Frank, Benjamin S. *No-Aging Diet*. New York: Dial, 1976.

*Fredericks, Carlton. *Eating Right for You*. New York: Grosset and Dunlap, 1972.

*——. *Look Younger/Feel Healthier*. New York: Grosset and Dunlap, 1977.

*——. *Psycho Nutrients*. New York: Grosset and Dunlap, 1976.

*Gomez, Joan and Gerch, Marvin J. *Dictionary of Symptoms*. New York: Stein and Day, 1968.

Goodhart, Robert S., and Shills, Maurice E. *Modern Nutrition in Health and Disease*. 5th ed. Philadelphia: Lea and Febiger, 1973.

*Graedon, Joe. *The People's Pharmacy*. New York: St. Martin's Press, 1976.

Guidelines for the Eradication of Iron Deficiency Anemia. New York: International Nutritional Anemia Consultative Group [INACG] 1976.

Guidelines for the Eradication of Vitamin-A Deficiency and Xerophthalmia. International Vitamin-A Consultative Group [IVACG].

Harper, Alfred E. "Recommended Dietary Allowances: Are They What We Think They Are?" *Journal of the American Dietetic Association* 64 [February 1974].

Holvey, David, ed. *The Merck Manual*. 12th ed. Rahway, N.J.: Merck and Co., 1972.

Howe, Phyllis S. *Basic Nutrition in Health and Disease*. 6th ed. Philadelphia: W.B. Saunders Co., 1976.

"How Nutritious Are Fast-Food Meals?" *Consumer Reports* [May 1975].

*Hunter, B.T. *The Natural Foods Primer*. New York: Simon and Schuster, 1972.

Index of Nutrition Education Materials. Washington, D.C.: Nutrition Foundation, 1977.

Journal of Applied Nutrition. International College of Applied Nutrition, La Habra, CA, 1974–76.

*Karelitz, Samuel. *When Your Child Is Ill*. New York: Random House, 1969.

Katz, Marcella. *Vitamins, Food, and Your Health*. Public Affairs Committee, 1971, 1975.*Kordel, L. *Health Through Nutrition*. New York: MacFadden-Bartell, 1971.

*Linde, Shirley. *The Whole Health Catalog*. New York: Rawson Associates Publishers, 1977.

*Lucas, Richard. *Nature's Medicines*. New York: Prentice-Hall, 1966.

*McGinnis, Terri. *The Well Cat Book*. New York: Random House-Book-works, 1975.

*———. *The Well Dog Book*. New York: Random House-Bookworks, 1974.

"Marijuana: The Health Question." *Consumer Reports* 40 [March 1975].

*Martin, Clement G. *Low Blood Sugar: The Hidden Menace of Hypoglycaemia*. New York: Arco Publishing Co., 1976.

Martin, Marvin. *Great Vitamin Mystery*. Rosemont, IL: National Dairy Council, 1978.

*Mayer, Jean. *A Diet for Living*. New York: David McKay, 1975.

Mitchell, Helen S. "Recommended Dietary Allowances Up to Date." *Journal of the American Dietetic Association* 64 [February 1974].

National Health Federation Bulletin. November, 1978.

National Research Council. *Recommended Dietary Allowances*. 8th ed. revised. Washington, DC: National Academy of Sciences, 1974.

National Research Council. *Toxicants Occurring Naturally in Foods*. 2nd ed. Washington, DC: National Academy of Sciences, 1973.

*Newbold, H.L. *Dr. Newbold's Revolutionary New Discovery About*

Weight Loss. New York: Rawson Associates Publishers, 1977.

*——. *Mega-Nutrients for Your Nerves*. New York: Peter H. Wyden, Publisher, 1978.

*Null, Gary. *The Natural Organic Beauty Book*. New York: Dell, 1972.

*Null, Gary and Steve. *The Complete Book of Nutrition*. New York: Dell. 1972.

Nutrition Almanac. New York: McGraw-Hill, 1973.

Nutrition — Applied Personally. La Habra, CA: International College of Applied Nutrition, 1978.

Nutrition Information Resources for the Whole Family. National Nutrition Education Clearing House, 1978.

Nutrition Labeling: How It Can Work for You. National Nutrition Consortium, American Dietetic Association, 1975.

Nutrition Source Book. Rosemont, IL: National Dairy Council, 1978.

*Passwater, Richard A. *Super nutrition*. New York: Dial, 1975.

*Pauling, Linus. *Vitamin C and the Commond Cold*. New York: Bantam Books, 1971.

Piltz, Albert. *How Your Body Uses Food*. Rosemont, IL: National Dairy Council, 1960.

*Pommery, Jean. *What to Do till the Veterinarian Comes*. Radnor, PA: Children Book Company, 1976.

"Present Knowledge in Nutrition." *Nutrition Reviews*. Nutrition Foundation, Inc., 1976.

*Rodale, J.I. *The Complete Book of Minerals for Health*. 4th ed. Emmaus, PA: Rodale Books, 1976.

*——. *The Encyclopedia of Common Diseases*. Emmaus, PA: Rodale Press, 1976.

*Rosenberg, Harold, and Feldzaman. A.N. *Doctor's Book of Vitamin Therapy: Megavitamins for Health*. New York: Putnam's 1974.

*Seamen, Barbara and Gideon. *Women and the Crisis in Sex Hormones*. New York: Rawson Associates Publishers, 1977.

*Shute, Wilfred E., and Taub, Harold J. *Vitamin E for Ailing and Healthy Hearts*. New York: Pyramid Books, 1976.

*Spock, Benjamin. *Baby and Child Care*. New York: Simon and Schuster, 1976.

"Too Much Sugar." *Consumer Reports* 43 [March 1978].

Underwood, Eric J. *Trace Elements in Human and Animal Nutrition*. 4th ed. New York: Academic Press, 1977.

United Nations. Food and Agriculture Organization. *Calorie Requirements, 1957, 1972*.

U.S. Department of Agriculture, *Amino Acid Content of Food* by M.L. Orr and B.K. Watt, 1957; rev. 1968.

U.S. Department of Agriculture. Consumer and Food Economics Institute, Agricultural Research Service. *Composition of Foods: Raw, Processed, Prepared* by Bernice K. Watt and Annabel L. Merrill, 1975.

U.S. Department of Agriculture. *Energy Value of Foods: Basis and*

Derivation by Annabel L. Merrill and Bernice K. Watt, 1973.

U.S. Department of Agriculture. *Nutritive Value of American Foods* by Catherine F. Adams, 1975.

U.S. Department of Health, Education and Welfare. *Consumer Health Education: A Directory*, 1975.

U.S. Department of Health, Education and Welfare. *Ten-State Nutrition Survey*. Washington, DC: U.S. Government Printing Office, 1968–70.

"The U.S. Food and Drug Administration: On Food and Drugs." *Consumer Reports* 38 [March 1973].

U.S. President's Council on Physical Fitness and Sports. *Exercise and Weight Control* by Robert E. Johnson, Urbana, IL: Univ. of Illinois Press, 1967.

U.S. Senate. Select Committee on Nutrition and Human Needs. *Diet and Killer Diseases with Press Reaction and Additional Information*. Washington, DC: U.S. Government Printing Office, 1977.

U.S. Senate. Select Committee on Nutrition and Human Needs. *National Nutrition Policy: Nutrition and the Consumer II*. Washington, DC: U.S. Government Printing Office, 1974.

"Vitamin-Mineral Safety, Toxicity and Misuse." *Journal of the American Dietetic Association*, 1978.

*Wade, Carlson. *Magic Minerals*. West Nyack, NY: Parker Publishing Co., 1967.

*——. *Miracle Protein*. West Nyack, NY: Parker Publishing Co., 1975.

*——. *Vitamin E: The Rejuvenation Vitamin*. New York: Award Books, 1970.

"Which Cereals Are Most Nutritious?" *Consumer Reports 40* [February 1975].

Williams, Roger, J. *Nutrition Against Disease*. New York: Pitman Publishers, 1971.

*Winter, Ruth. *A Consumer's Dictionary of Food Additives*. New York: Crown, 1978.

*Young, Klein, Beyer. *Recreational Drugs*. New York: Macmillan, 1977.

*Yudkin, John. *Sweet and Dangerous*. New York: Peter H. Wyden, 1972.

Index

229

cola 130, 189–91, 207, 221
cold pressed ointments 137
colds 48, 54, 173, 195
cold sores 160, 180
colitis 62, 173
collagen 30, 48, 213
colon *see* large intestine
comfrey 208
concentration 42, 102
congenital achlorhydria 141
conjunctivitis 54
connective tissue 65
constipation 93, 111, 114, 115, 121,
  142, 160–1, 167, 173
convulsions 108, 220
cooking
  to destroy vitamin content 50, 66
  to maintain vitamin content 132–3
copper 75–6, 79, 106, 115, 128, 205,
  208, 214, 221, 222
copper pots 132
corn syrup 198–9
corticosteroids 195
cortisone 63, 130, 138, 195, 196, 221
cosmetics, what's in natural 210–12
cot death 48
Coumadin 219
cravings, possible meaning of 129–32
creatine 107
cuts 161
cyanide 46
cyanocobalamin *see* vitamin B12
cysteine 95, 106, 111, 167
cystine 95, 106, 107
Cytochrome-C 152

Dalmane 70
damiana 164
dancers, regimen for 153
dandruff 87
dark-skinned people 55
Darvon 182
deficiency diseases See specific
  Vitamin or disease
  hoq to test for 118–19
  possible warning signs 119–29
dehydration 30, 93, 94, 152
dementia 181
dental postoperative pain 37
dentists and dental hygienists 77, 184–
  5
deodorants 90, 113
depressants 191

depression 76, 81, 99, 105, 106, 108,
  143, 177, 181–3, 222
dermatitis 30, 47, 128, 209, 218
dextrose 198
DHEA (dehydroepiandrosterone) 214
diabetes 39, 41, 50, 74, 92, 107, 110,
  115, 130, 151, 174, 175, 199, 219, 220
diarrhoea 35, 63, 64, 85, 111, 121, 142,
  173, 181, 218
dicalcium phosphate 25, 30
Dicumarol 220
diet drugs 108, 109
dieting 77, 93, 198–203
diets 200–03
digestion
  poor 115, 195
  process 17, 37, 73, 82, 93
digestive enzymes *see* enzymes
digestive system 17–20, 63, 114
digoxin 222
diluents 24–5, 30
Dilantin 60, 222
dinner 202–3
  high-pep supplements 150, 215–16
dirt, children eating 132
disease
  prevention 7, 79
  resistance to 104
disintegration 25
diuretic(s) 30, 36, 40, 56, 81, 112, 164,
  178, 220
  potassium loss and 86, 87, 130, 195
diverticulosis 114
dizziness 66, 83, 102, 121, 172, 200
DL-phenylalanine (DLPA) 100–1
DNA 30, 91, 190, 203, 213–14
  basic vitamin-mineral RNA-DNA
    programme 214
  -RNA supplements 7, 59, 148, 149,
    213–14, 222
doctors, regimen for 155
dolomite 24, 72, 81, 193
Dong Quai 178
dopamine 99
dream recall 41
drinkers, regimen for 157; *see also*
  alcohol
drug(s)
  alternatives to 191, 194
  caffeine in common 190–1
  that induce vitamin loss, chart of 196–7
  vs. vitamins 189–203
  withdrawal 189

231

236